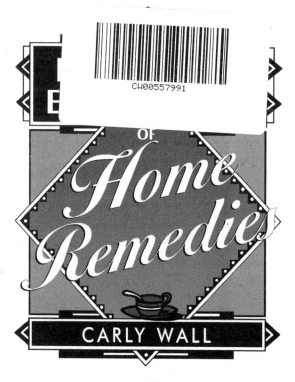

THE LITTLE ENCYCLOPEDIA

OF

Home Remedies

CARLY WALL

Sterling Publishing Co., Inc.
New York

Edited and arranged by Jeanette Green

Library of Congress Cataloging-in-Publication Data

Wall, Carly, 1960–
    The little giant encyclopedia of home remedies/Carly Wall.
        p. cm.
    Includes index.
    ISBN 0-8069-9815-6
    1. Naturopathy—Encyclopedias. 2. Materia medica,
Vegetable—Encyclopedias. 3. Herbs—Therapeutic use—
Encyclopedias. I. Title.
    RZ433.W35 2000
    615.5'35—dc21   99-012496

1 3 5 7 9 10 8 6 4 2
Published by Sterling Publishing Co., Inc.
387 Park Avenue South, New York, New York 10016
© 2000 by Carly Wall
Distributed in Canada by Sterling Publishing
%Canadian Manda Group, One Atlantic Avenue, Suite 105
Toronto, Ontario, Canada M6K 3E7
Distributed in Great Britain and Europe by Cassell PLC
Wellington House, 125 Strand, London WC2R 0BB, England
Distributed in Australia by Capricorn Link (Australia) Pty Ltd.
P.O. Box 6651, Baulkham Hills, Business Centre, NSW 2153,
Australia
Manufactured in the United States of America
All rights reserved
ISBN 0-8069-9815-6

CONTENTS

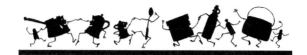

INTRODUCTION

The fun of making your own home remedies is that you get to save money, and you can also get that warm, satisfying feeling of being independent every time you mix up a batch of what you need at the moment. Another plus is that you don't have to drop what you're doing to run off to the nearest market or "super" store. And too, there's always that feeling of being linked to the past—remembering how Grandma mixed up her famous recipes to soothe our skinned knees or showing us how she made and used her potpourris.

Making your own home remedies puts you in charge of the ingredients that go into your own creations. Perhaps that's why Grandma often had a smile on her face. She never had to wonder if something had been chemically adulterated or contained only what the label said. There's nothing better than freshly picked herbs from your own herb patch or honey from a neighbor's hive. Best of all, you'll be the one in the neighborhood who gives the best gifts from the heart and hearth—your own kitchen.

Have fun—I surely have. I've mixed recipes that didn't quite make the grade, but turned out useful for something else. Some were disasters altogether, but I've left those out of this book! I have a few favorite recipes that I use over and over. You'll find these favorites inside light gray boxes.

I love to try out new recipes and hope you do, too. Here are the best old-time recipes I've collected over the years. I hope they bring you as much joy and practical healing as they have me.

—Carly Wall

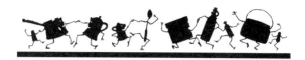

Part 1
SIMPLE ILLS

In this part, you'll find remedies for symptom relief from the common cold, flu, coughs, congestion, scrapes, cuts, wounds, burns, skin irritations, and more.

These tonics, teas, rubs, and other remedies contain herbs and other natural ingredients. In general, they're safer than most over-the-counter drugs. Check for allergies and only use them as directed.

You'll find easy relief from insect bites,

poison ivy and poison oak, athlete's foot, ringworm, and fungal infections. Discover traditional treatments for styes, boils, warts, and moles.

Create your own homemade remedies for digestive upsets, like constipation, diarrhea, gastritis, indigestion, and heartburn, as well as ulcers and stomach pain, nausea, and motion sickness.

Tonics will help you feel healthy. You'll find symptom relief from arthritis, gout, and muscle aches, as well as sinus, migraine, or allergy headaches.

COLDS & FLU

Many cold and flu symptoms are similar. Americans typically contract two or three colds a year. Flu season usually begins in the fall, when children return to school.

Cold symptoms include watery eyes, headaches, fever, chills, muscle aches, nose and throat irritations, and temporary loss of smell and taste. A cold attacks the upper respiratory tract and causes sneezing, coughing, and difficulty breathing. The mucus helps rid the body of infection.

Influenza, what we commonly call flu, is an acute viral infection of the respiratory tract. It is highly contagious and easily spread by coughing and sneezing. Symptoms of flu are chills, high fever, sore throat, headache, abdominal pain, hoarseness, cough, and enlarged lymph nodes. Also vomiting, diarrhea, and weak or aching arms, legs, and back are common. Complications like pneumonia, sinus infections, and ear infections can develop.

Stomach flu, or gastroenteritis, on the other hand, can have a variety of causes, like food poisoning, drug sensitivity, allergy, reaction to certain viruses, or overindulgence in alcohol.

Colds

Chicken Soup

Grandma was right. Chicken soup can help clear the lungs, and it promotes perspiration, which can help rid the body of toxins. Eat a hot bowl of this soup, and then wrap yourself under a heavy quilt for a nap. The hot soup soothes irritated throats and eases you to sleep.

Chicken & Herb Soup

  4 cups chicken stock
  5 garlic cloves, minced
  1½ teaspoons dried dill weed
  1½ teaspoons dried parsley
  1½ teaspoons dried thyme
  ½ teaspoon cayenne pepper
  1 cup noodles (optional)

Heat the chicken stock and garlic to boiling. Add the dill weed, parsley, thyme, and cayenne pepper. Also add 1 cup or more of noodles, if desired. Cook until the noodles are done.

  This makes a healthful soup to enjoy anytime, but all ingredients, except for the noodles, contribute to boosting the immune system and getting rid of viruses and other germs.

Thyme Congestion Mist

1 tablespoon dried thyme or eucalyptus
boiling water

Put the dried thyme or eucalyptus in a
heat-resistant bowl. Pour boiling water
over the herb. Tent a towel over your head
and the bowl so that you can breathe in
the vapors for 6 to 8 minutes. This mist
clears the head and stuffy noses.

Thyme is a good germ killer. Eucalyptus
is great for bronchial congestion and excess
mucus.

Hyssop & Mullein Tincture for Coughs

dried hyssop
dried mullein
vodka

Combine equal amounts of dried hyssop and mullein in a Mason jar. Cover completely with vodka. Let the herbs steep in a sunny window for 2 weeks. Strain.

For coughs, put 30 drops of this tincture in ½ cup of water and drink.

You can drink up to 3 cups per day. This tincture is helpful for soothing and relaxing the lungs and bronchial tubes. It helps ease persistent coughing fits associated with viral infections.

Lemonade Cold Cure

  2 tablespoons lemon juice concentrate
  ¾ cup water
  1 teaspoon dried comfrey leaves

Bring the lemon juice, water, and comfrey leaves to a boil. Remove it from heat, strain, and drink at bedtime. Be sure to go to bed and cover yourself up.

  This brew will bring on a sweat. The comfrey is good at breaking up colds and is one of the rare plant sources for vitamin B_{12}.

Honeycomb Cure

Chewing honeycomb keeps the nose open and dry.

Honey Milk for Colds
   1 cup milk
   1 tablespoon honey

Heat the milk and add the honey. Stir well. Drink the honey milk while it is still warm. This recipe will help you sleep more comfortably when you have a cold.

Lemon Juice & Honey Gargle
   2 teaspoons honey
   1 teaspoon lemon juice
   1 cup warm water

Mix honey, lemon juice, and warm water. Use this gargle at least twice a day. Honey and lemon juice soothe and act as antiseptics and soothe sore throats when gargled.

Onion Cure

  4 large onions
  honey

Clean the onions, and cut them into
chunks. Add to a saucepan and cover with
water. Simmer until the onions are softened. Strain out and keep the juice. Add
equal amounts of honey to the juice. Mix
well. Take several tablespoons at bedtime
to help break up colds and coughs.

Flu

Spicy Flu Tea

1 teaspoon powdered cinnamon
1 teaspoon powdered ginger
6 cardamom seeds
2 cups boiling water

Add the cinnamon, ginger, and cardamom seeds to the boiling water. Reduce heat to simmer and let simmer 20 minutes, covered. Drink 2 cups of tea in 1 day.

Cinnamon kills viruses. Ginger relieves nausea and boosts the immune system. Cardamom reduces body aches.

Herbal Intestinal Flu Relief

   dried chamomile flowers
   dried catnip leaves
   dried peppermint leaves
   1 cup boiling water
   honey (optional)

Use equal amounts chamomile, catnip, and peppermint. Mix well. Put in a Mason jar and seal. Be sure to label.

To use, place a heaping teaspoon in a tea ball in boiling water. Steep for 6 minutes. Strain. Add honey and sip. This tea can be taken every hour until flu symptoms abate.

Chamomile flowers settle an upset stomach. Catnip leaves calm nerves and settle the stomach. Peppermint leaves help relieve nausea and promote digestion.

Feverfew Flu Pain Relief

   1 teaspoon dried lavender buds
   2 fresh or ⅛ teaspoon dried feverfew leaves
   pinch nutmeg
   1 cinnamon stick
   1 cup boiling water
   honey (optional)

Pour boiling water over the lavender buds, feverfew leaves, nutmeg, and cinnamon stick. Let steep 5 minutes. Strain. Add honey to taste. Drink up to 2 cups per day before naps or at bedtime.

   This tea will help relieve aches and pains associated with flu.

Coughs

Although coughs help rid the lungs of phlegm and congestion, anyone who has stayed awake all night coughing knows how disturbing a cough can be. Sleep is vital to healing.

If you have a serious, lingering cold, bronchitis, or pneumonia, some coughing fits may even seem so painful and severe as to threaten to break ribs. Of course, you'll want to consult a physician for a cold that doesn't go away in a week or two.

Folk remedies for coughs and colds abound. Here are a few we've collected from the Shakers, American Indians, and others.

Traditional cough syrups and drops often use horehound (*Marrubium vulgare*) flowers or leaves. These horehound recipes help reduce congestion. Horehound also acts as an antiseptic. The Shakers, famous for their horehound cough syrups, also made a hard horehound candy for use as cough drops during long, cold winters.

Horehound Cough Syrup

   1 tablespoon horehound
   1 cup boiling water
   2 tablespoons honey

Add two parts honey to one part of strong horehound tea to make a good cough syrup.

Horehound Cough Drops

horehound leaves and flowers
1 cup boiling water
3¾ cups sugar
1½ cups light corn syrup

Make a strong tea of horehound leaves and
flowers. Add 1 cup tea to 3¾ cups sugar
and 1½ cups light corn syrup. Mix in a
large saucepan, stirring over medium heat
until the sugar dissolves.

Next, bring the mixture to a boil, without
stirring, until the temperature on a candy
thermometer reaches 310º F (154º C) or
drops of syrup form hard, brittle threads in
cold water. Remove from heat. Pour into
ungreased molds or onto a lightly greased
cookie sheet.

Cool; then unmold or break the candy
into pieces. Pieces can be dusted with

powdered sugar to keep them from sticking together. Store them in airtight containers or plastic bags. This recipe makes a little over 2 pounds (about 1 kg) of cough drops.

Irish Cough Syrup
  2 cups good Irish whiskey
  ¼ cup lemon juice
  2 teaspoons aniseed
  ½ cup sugar

Mix the Irish whiskey, lemon juice, aniseed, and sugar. Boil the mixture for 6 minutes. Strain out the seeds and bottle. Take 1 teaspoon as needed.

Pine-Bark Cough Syrup

¼ cup dried red clover blossoms
¼ cup dried coltsfoot leaves
¼ cup dried mullein leaves
¼ cup licorice root pieces
1 cup white-pine bark
1 cup water
2 cups "real" maple syrup

Put the clover blossoms, coltsfoot leaves, mullein leaves, licorice root pieces, and white-pine bark in a pan with the water. Place the pan on low heat for 4 hours. Stir every so often. Do not boil the mixture since the herbs will lose their effectiveness. Strain; simply squeeze out the liquid. Add the liquid to the maple syrup. Mix, bottle, and refrigerate.

To use: take 1 teaspoon of this cough syrup every 2 hours or as needed.

Oswego Tea Cough Remedy

  2 teaspoons fresh or 1 teaspoon dried
   Oswego tea leaves
  1 cup boiling water
  honey (optional)

Place fresh or dried Oswego tea leaves in boiling water. Cover and steep 5 minutes. Add honey to taste. Sip up to 3 cups per day as needed.

Oswego tea is also known as Indian nettle or *Monarda didyma*. The herb, often used by Native Americans, contains antiseptic properties and helps clear congestion and respiratory infections.

Wild Cherry Cough Syrup

4 tablespoons wild-cherry bark
4 tablespoons dried New Jersey tea leaves
  and seeds (*Ceanothus americanus*)
4 tablespoons dried mullein
2 cups boiling water
3 pounds (1.35 kg) brown sugar
½ cup lemon juice

Put the wild-cherry bark, New Jersey tea leaves and seeds, and mullein in the boiling water. Turn down the heat, cover, and simmer for 20 minutes. Strain. Add the brown sugar and lemon juice. Bring to boil again and boil until the mixture becomes a thick syrup. Bottle. Take 1 tablespoon as needed.

Mom's Favorite Cherry Cough Syrup

2 cups (1 pint) cherries
½ lemon, sliced
water
2 cups honey

Place cherries and lemon in a pan and just cover with water. Bring to a boil. Add the honey. Simmer until the cherries are soft. Strain and bottle.

Keep this cough syrup in the refrigerator and give 2 tablespoons as needed for coughs.

Garlic Elixir for Coughs

4 cloves garlic
2 pieces ginger root
1 cup water
1 cup honey

Pour the water into a pan and add the garlic and ginger root. Boil for 20 minutes. Remove from heat. Strain. Add honey and mix well.

Take 1 tablespoon for coughs and sore throats.

Chest Rubs

Peppermint & Rosemary Chest Rub

   3 tablespoons strong, double-strength
     peppermint tea
   1 tablespoon strong, double-strength rose-
     mary tea
   4 tablespoons dark molasses
   2 tablespoons olive oil

Use 2 tea bags and ½ cup boiling water to make strong peppermint tea. Steep for 10 minutes. Do the same for the strong rosemary tea. Combine the molasses, olive oil, peppermint tea, and rosemary tea and mix well.

   Take 1 teaspoonful before each meal. This old-time remedy for deep chest colds has been praised as a sure cure.

Camphor & Eucalyptus Chest Rub

  1 fluid ounce olive oil
  ½ teaspoon grated beeswax
  30 drops eucalyptus essential oil
  40 drops camphor essential oil
  15 drops peppermint essential oil

Warm olive oil, add grated beeswax, and gently warm until melted. Remove from heat, and then stir in the eucalyptus, camphor, and peppermint essential oils. Pour into a container.

When you have a cold, this ointment, rubbed on the chest, will help ease breathing and reduce congestion.

Fevers

Lemon Fever-Reducing Tea
  1 whole lemon
  1 teaspoon dried comfrey
  1 teaspoon dried thyme
  1 cup boiling water

Chop the lemon into small pieces. Add the comfrey, thyme, and lemon to a saucepan with boiling water. Simmer 5 minutes. Strain and drink while hot—just not hot enough to burn your tongue.

Room Spray

Spicy Antiviral Room & Air Scent
  1 teaspoon whole cloves
  1 teaspoon cinnamon
  1 teaspoon lemon peel
  ½ cup apple-cider vinegar
  ½ cup water

Put the whole cloves, cinnamon, lemon peel, apple-cider vinegar, and water in a pan and simmer on the stove or in a potpourri burner. Be careful that the liquid doesn't simmer away and burn the pan.

Whenever colds or flu strike a household, germs abound. This recipe will cleanse the air and make everything more antiseptic. To disinfect surfaces, strain and let the mixture cool. Simply dip a clean rag into the solution and wring it out. Then wipe down sinks, telephones, toilets, and more.

WOUNDS & CUTS

Here are some recipes for wounds and cuts that help soothe and heal broken skin. Many have natural antiseptic properties. Consult a physician for large wounds.

These recipes are not intended for use on burns, since many contain oils. Always avoid oils and butters when treating burns. Please see the section on Burns on pp. 52–59.

Balm of Gilead Bud Tincture

½ cup balm of Gilead buds
whiskey

Bruise or nick the balm of Gilead buds with a knife. In a pint (2-cup or about 500-ml) jar, put the balm of Gilead buds and add whiskey to cover. Seal the jar and shake it every day for a week. After a week, the tincture will be ready to use.

Apply the balm with a cotton ball to cuts, wounds, or scrapes. Balm of Gilead buds are healing and help ease pain.

Sweet Woodruff & Chamomile Tincture

dried sweet woodruff
dried chamomile blooms
sunflower oil or olive oil

Fill a pint (2-cup or about 500-ml) jar half
with dried sweet woodruff and half with
dried chamomile blooms. Cover these with
a good-quality sunflower oil or olive oil.
Let steep in a sunny window for 2 weeks;
shake every day. Strain. Apply to wounds
with a cotton ball or clean cloth.

Sweet woodruff has a long history as a
wound healer. Chamomile acts as an anti-
inflammatory that's helpful for shingles, as
well as for infections and wounds. You
cannot miss having this on hand.

Mallow Wound Wash

   ¾ cup chopped mallow root
   ½ cup mallow leaves
   4 cups boiling water

Add the mallow root and leaves to the
boiling water. Let steep until cool. Strain.
Use this as a cleansing wash for inflamed
wounds.

Plantain Poultice

   ½ cup fresh plantain leaves
   ½ cup water
   honey

Bring water to boil and add plantain
leaves. Reduce heat to simmer for 10 minutes. Strain. Add equal amounts of honey
to the mixture. Smear this poultice on the
inflamed wound and bandage it overnight.

Just Honey

  honey

Honey, used alone, is naturally healing. It helps cleanse wounds of bacteria and helps prevent scarring. Physicians once smeared honey on wounds, covering lightly with a bandage. The dressing was changed daily and more honey added.

Honey Salve

  2 teaspoons cod-liver oil
  2 teaspoons honey

Mix the cod-liver oil and honey thoroughly and apply the salve to the affected area. Cover lightly with a bandage. Apply more salve with a fresh bandage daily until the wound heals. This honey salve is especially healing for minor cuts.

Minor Skin Wound Balm

  ⅓ cup dried calendula blossoms
  ⅓ cup dried comfrey leaves
  ⅓ cup dried thyme
  1 cup olive oil
  2 tablespoons vitamin E oil
  4 tablespoons melted beeswax

Mix the calendula blossoms, comfrey leaves, and thyme well. Pack the dried material into a jar and cover it with olive oil. Add vitamin E oil as a preservative. Place the jar in sunny window for 2 weeks. Strain. Melt the beeswax, remove it from heat, and stir in the strained oil. Mix well. Pour the skin balm into decorative jars with lids. This recipe makes about 1 cup or 8 fluid ounces (240 ml).

Keep this wound balm on hand for emergencies. Apply it to minor skin scrapes, wounds, or irritations. Calendula acts as an anti-inflammatory, and thyme acts as an antiseptic. Comfrey promotes cell renewal and speeds healing.

***

Goldenseal Wash

1 heaping teaspoon powdered goldenseal
1 heaping teaspoon powdered myrrh
2 cups boiling water

Steep the goldenseal and myrrh in the water for 15 minutes. Wash the wound with this water when it is cool to the touch.

This wash cleanses and heals wounds.

Goldenseal Liniment

  2 tablespoons powdered goldenseal
  ¼ cup (2 ounces or 58 g) powdered myrrh
  4 cups rubbing alcohol

Mix the goldenseal, myrrh, and alcohol.
Allow the mixture to steep for 1 week,
shaking it every day. Strain. Apply the liniment with a clean cloth or cotton ball
three to four times a day. This herbal liniment relieves soreness and pain and helps
heal.

❧

Geranium Cuts & Abrasions Remedy

  geranium leaves

For small cuts or wounds, pick some leaves
of the common geranium plant. Bruise
them and rub them over the wound; it
should heal in no time.

Wound-Healing Green Potion

¼ cup dried or ½ cup fresh comfrey leaves
¼ cup dried or ½ cup fresh yarrow leaves
¾ cup peanut oil
1 tablespoon melted beeswax

In a saucepan, cover the comfrey leaves and yarrow leaves with peanut oil and heat gently, just to warm, for 30 minutes. Strain. Beat in the melted beeswax. Pour into short containers with lids. Rub the cream on clean wounds, scratches, or cuts.

Keep the cream refrigerated. The peanut oil will harden to a thick cream when kept cold. It should stay fresh up to a year.

Calendula Relief Cream

   1 cup olive oil
   ¾ cup calendula flower petals
   4 teaspoons grated beeswax

Warm the olive oil in a saucepan. Add the calendula flower petals and let steep for 30 minutes. Strain. For every cup of olive oil, add the grated beeswax. Heat until the beeswax melts. Mix completely and pour into little jars. Seal tight and keep refrigerated.

   Spread on affected areas as needed. This cream will help soothe burns and reduce inflammation.

Healing Lavender Cream

  2 cups powdered lavender buds
  ¾ cup melted vegetable shortening
  1 tablespoon melted beeswax
  1 teaspoon vitamin E oil

Powder the dried lavender buds in a blender or food processor. Place the shortening in saucepan and heat until melted. Add powdered lavender. Let steep on low heat for 30 minutes. Strain. Add beeswax to the shortening and allow it to melt over low heat. Mix well. To lengthen shelf life, add the vitamin E oil. Pour into small jars.

  This cream can help heal wounds and inflammations as well as help prevent infections. It is good for scrapes and cuts, especially for children. This is a wonderfully mild, yet healing, ointment.

BURNS

Please Note: These burn remedies are for minor, first-degree burns. Second- and third-degree burns require immediate medical attention. Generally, it's best to avoid using butters and oils on burns. Also, avoid heat.

Whenever you get a burn, dunk it as quickly as possible in cold water. You want to cool the burn down as soon as you can to minimize damage to skin. Immediately reach for aloe vera or ice to soothe skin and cool the burn. Aloe vera also has healing properties.

Aloe Vera & Honey Sunburn Relief

¼ cup dried calendula flowers
¼ cup dried lavender buds
¼ cup dried peppermint
¼ cup aloe-vera juice
¼ cup honey
2 cups water

Place water in a saucepan and bring to a boil. Turn down the heat. Add the calendula flowers, lavender buds, and peppermint, gently heating on low for 10 minutes. Strain. Add the aloe-vera juice and honey and mix well.

Pour the mixture into a spray bottle, and spray the affected area freely several times a day. This spray helps relieve the heating and cooling effects of sunburn.

Vinegar Sunburn Relief

apple-cider vinegar

Apple-cider vinegar is very soothing and healing. Soak a clean cloth in vinegar and apply it to the sunburned area. The vinegar will soon take away the pain. Use when needed.

Yarrow & Potato Sunburn Relief

3 large potatoes
water
handful white yarrow flowers and leaves

Slice the potatoes and cover them with water. Add the handful of white yarrow blooms and leaves. Boil 5 minutes. Cool. Strain. Soak a cloth in the liquid, squeeze out a little, and apply as a loose bandage on the sunburn. This helps reduce pain.

Honey Sunburn Lotion

½ cup olive oil
2 tablespoons honey
½ cup apple-cider vinegar

Warm the olive oil gently and blend in the honey and vinegar. Let cool. Apply liberally as needed. Keep on hand in the summer.

Sunburn Lavender Spritz

¼ cup olive oil
¼ cup dried lavender buds
2 tablespoons vitamin E oil

Gently warm the olive oil and add the lavender buds. Let warm gently for 15 minutes. Strain. Cool and add the vitamin E oil. Place in a small spray bottle and keep on hand to spritz sunburn. This healing spritz prevents scars, and lavender will dull the pain.

Avoid using oils on burns. Here are a few simple remedies.

Honey: Apply honey as soon as possible after a minor burn. Honey speeds healing and takes away pain.

Aloe Vera: Another easy and quick remedy involves the aloe-vera plant. I keep a plant growing on my kitchen windowsill. That way, when someone gets a minor kitchen burn, I can break off a leaf quickly and apply the soothing gel right to the affected area. Just squeeze out the juice and smooth it on. In seconds, the stinging pain is gone.

The plant is easy to grow; it doesn't need much water or attention.

Wild & Woolly Burn Remedy

    handful fresh chickweed (*Stellaria media*)
    handful fresh comfrey (*Symphytum officinale*)
    ice water

Place clean, rinsed chickweed and comfrey in a blender. Add a little ice water and grind to form a green paste. Apply to burns. This burn remedy is antiseptic and healing to the skin.

Chamomile Bags for Burns

    1 to 8 chamomile tea bags
    1 cup boiling water
    ice water

Dunk a chamomile tea bag in boiling water. Squeeze out slightly and dunk the tea bag in ice water. Apply the cool bags to affected areas. The soothing chamomile helps ease pain.

Chamomile Bath: Place 5 to 8 tea bags in 1 cup boiling water. Steep for 5 minutes. Squeeze the bags out. Add this liquid to a cool bath.

❧

Lavender & Chamomile Burn Wash

½ cup lavender flower buds
½ cup chamomile flowers
2 cups boiling water

Pour the boiling water over the lavender flower buds and chamomile flowers. Let the mixture steep for 5 to 8 minutes or until cool. Add ice. Dip a cloth into the cool mixture, wring it out slightly, and lay the cloth over the burned area. Keep the cloth in place until the cloth feels warm. Repeat and keep repeating until the pain subsides.

Calendula Flower Poultice

dry calendula flowers
water

Dry calendula flowers in quantity to keep them on hand. In a blender, powder the petals and store them in a closed jar. Label the jar so that you'll know what it is. When needed, take a small amount of the powder and add water to form a paste. Apply this to burns; then cover the burn with a loose cotton-gauze bandage.

Slippery-Elm Paste

3 tablespoons powdered slippery elm bark
hot water

For this traditional remedy, use powdered slippery-elm bark and add enough hot water to form a paste. When this cools, apply the paste to the burned area.

INSECT BITES

See also household and personal Insect
Repellants on pp. 390–406.

Insect Repellant & Bite Relief

¼ cup olive oil
5 drops cedarwood essential oil
5 drops camphor tincture
2 drops citronella essential oil

Mix the olive oil, cedarwood essential oil,
camphor tincture, and citronella essential
oil well. Rub on the skin to prevent mosquito bites and bites from other insects.
Also, apply to bites to take out the sting
and soreness.

This was adapted from an old Amish
recipe.

Lavender Sting & Bite Remedy

   lavender essential oil

For bee or wasp stings, make sure the stinger is removed. Apply lavender essential oil full strength. Wait a few minutes and apply again.

   Lavender essential oil can also prevent infections from bites. Use it for a variety of bites and stings. It is an all-purpose healer, and it is the only essential oil, besides tea tree, that you can apply full-strength to the skin without dilution. (For sensitive skin, however, tea tree may need to be diluted.)

   Lavender will help relieve hornet, wasp, or bee stings as well as spider, chigger, mosquito, or fly bites.

Chamomile Bag for Bites

  1 chamomile tea bag
  ½ cup boiling water
  ice water

Insect bites and stings cause itching and
swelling. Chamomile soothes and helps
reduce the inflammation. Dip a chamomile
tea bag into boiling water. Squeeze out and
dunk into ice water. Squeeze out excess
water and apply the tea bag to the bite.

Wasp-Sting Relief

Apple-cider vinegar is good for this. Soak
a cotton ball in apple-cider vinegar and
apply to the sting as often as needed. It
should take away the pain.

Healing Paste

baking soda
water or vinegar

For a painful bite, take a pinch of baking
soda and place it in your palm. Now add a
few drops of water to form a paste. Apply
this paste to the insect bite, and it should
stop the itching and pain.

Or use equal parts of baking soda and
vinegar to make a paste.

Onion Poultice

fresh onion

A freshly cut onion draws out the "poison"
if applied to a bee sting or other insect
bite.

Basil Bee-Sting Remedy

crushed basil stem and leaves

Basil is the best herb available to relieve any stings you may get. Always have some growing in your garden. That way, when you get an insect sting in the summer, you'll have fresh leaves to grab when you need them.

Break off pieces of the stem and leaves and crush them to release the juice. Apply this basil-juice poultice to the sting. In minutes, the pain and swelling will be gone.

Herbal Bee-Sting Poultice

  echinacea, fennel, hyssop, or marjoram stem
  and leaves

The herbs echinacea, fennel, hyssop, and marjoram can be used for bee stings. Break off pieces of the stem and leaves and crush them to release the juice. Apply an herb-juice poultice to the sting.

  While these herbs work, basil seems to be the most effective bee-sting remedy.

Sting Tenderizer

  meat tenderizer
  water

Many people swear by using meat tenderizer on stings or bites. Just make a paste with a little water and apply it to the skin.

SKIN IRRITATIONS

These remedies are all intended for topical (external) use on the skin to soothe irritations and help heal.

To powder herbs, you can use a mortar and pestle, food processor, or blender. Of course, it would be best to reserve a small food processor or blender for the purpose. You want to avoid using it for food. Not all herbs and oils are edible.

Use cold-pressed, cold-processed oils. Castor beans are poisonous but the oil, if properly prepared, reportedly is not.

Poison Ivy & Poison Oak
If you've accidentally rubbed against poison ivy or poison oak, immediately wash off the area with a strong hand soap, like the kind used in many public-park buildings. This may prevent you from getting a rash.

Jewelweed Poison Ivy & Oak Remedy

2 cups jewelweed stems and leaves
4 cups water

Add the jewelweed stems and leaves to the water. Bring to a boil. Remove from heat, cover, and let steep for 10 minutes. Strain. When cool, apply this tea to the poison-ivy or poison-oak rash and other affected areas.

This is the best "cure" for poison ivy or poison oak. Jewelweed often grows near the offending poison-ivy and poison-oak vines.

Sassafras-Root Bath

sassafras roots
water

Sassafras roots can ease suffering from a poison-ivy rash. Use clean roots, added to a small pot of water, to make a strong tea. Bring the water and roots to a boil and reduce the heat to simmer. Cover and simmer for 30 minutes. Strain. Add the strong tea to your bathwater. Soak in the bath for 20 minutes.

Valerian Root Tincture

¼ cup valerian root
2 cups vodka

Steep the valerian root in the vodka for 2 weeks. Strain and bottle. This tincture will keep indefinitely. Use cotton balls to apply to affected areas.

Boils

A boil is an inflammation and swelling that results from infection in a skin gland that forms a hard core and pus. Anyone who has had a boil knows how irritating and unsightly it can be. Here are some useful remedies for getting rid of them.

Linseed Paste

raw linseed oil
honey
flour

Use equal parts of raw linseed oil and honey. Add enough flour to make a paste. Apply to the boil several times a day.

Pork-Rind Poultice

 pork rind or bacon fat

Apply a piece of pork rind or bacon fat to
the boil and cover it with a bandage
overnight. This helps draw the infection
out. This traditional remedy is very effective.

Hot Tea-Tree Compress

 1 cup hot water
 ¼ cup salt
 ¼ cup Epsom salts
 3 to 6 drops tea-tree essential oil

Use a hot compress to draw out boils. Soak
a cloth in hot water in which the table salt
and Epsom salts have been dissolved. Add
a few drops of tea-tree essential oil. Apply
the warm compress to the boil three times
a day.

Styes

Black-Tea Stye Remedy
  black tea bag
  water

Moisten a black tea bag and apply as a compress over the eye. Let the compress stay on for 15 to 20 minutes. Do this twice a day until you feel relief.

Warts & Moles

Raw Turnip or Potato: Rub a raw turnip or potato over the area once or twice a day until you achieve desired results.
Tea-Tree Essential Oil: Apply a drop of tea-tree essential oil to the wart daily.

Wart & Mole Removal

  cold-pressed, cold-processed castor oil
  baking soda

The best method for removing warts or
moles is to rub castor oil into the area
every day until it disappears. Use only
cold-pressed, cold-processed castor oil.

  Or make a paste with castor oil and baking soda. Apply the paste to the wart and
cover it with a bandage. Apply fresh for 3
days or longer or until the mole or wart
comes off.

❧

  This preparation works, but it must be
used cautiously. Use castor oil topically
(externally) for the wart or mole you want
to remove. Do not heat or warm castor oil.

Eczema

Eczema can range from a little redness to a rash to raw, oozing, infected skin. Allergy, whether topical or internal (from foods eaten, for instance), faulty nutrition, or a weakened immune system are often the culprits. However, check with a physician if the eczema persists, since there may be another, perhaps more serious, cause or disease of which this is merely a symptom.

Eczema Remedy

  handful sheep sorrel leaves or strawberry
    leaves
  2 cups boiling water

Put a handful of sheep sorrel leaves or strawberry leaves into boiling water. Remove from heat and let steep for 15 minutes. Strain and apply the wash to areas affected with eczema.

Lemon & Peanut Oil Skin Treatment

¼ cup peanut oil
48 drops lemon essential oil

A good eczema remedy combines peanut oil and lemon essential oil. To the peanut oil, add the lemon essential oil. Mix well. Apply to the affected area(s) before bed.

The peanut oil dilutes the essential oil while helping the skin absorb it. Oils also aid the skin's retention of moisture, making the area feel less "raw."

Caution: Avoid sunlight to the area when using this oil.

Rashes & Chapped Skin

Chamomile for Diaper Rash

  2 chamomile tea bags
  1 cup boiling water

Add the chamomile tea bags to the boiling water. Steep until the water is just warm to the touch. Remove the tea bags. Apply to baby's bottom with a cotton ball.

Herbal Powder for Heat & Diaper Rash

  2 tablespoons cornstarch
  2 tablespoons powdered lavender buds
  2 tablespoons powdered chamomile blossoms

To the cornstarch, add the powdered lavender buds and powdered chamomile blossoms. Blend well. Powder this lavender-chamomile blend on skin with heat or diaper rash.

Watermelon Prickly-Heat Remedy

watermelon rind

For prickly-heat rash, rub a watermelon rind over the rash and let it dry.

✺

Rose Skin Lotion

   1 cup rose petals
   1 cup peanut oil
   ½ cup olive oil

Add the rose petals to the peanut oil. Let steep in a sunny window for 2 weeks. Strain. Mix the olive oil into the steeped rose solution, and place it in a squeeze bottle.

Add 1 tablespoon or more to bathwater. This lotion soothes and moisturizes rough or chapped skin.

Chapped Lips & Skin Treatment

½ cup sesame oil
¼ cup calendula petals
¼ cup St.-John's-wort leaves

To the sesame oil, add calendula petals and St.-John's-wort leaves. Gently warm the oil and add the herbs. Remove from heat and cover. Let steep for 30 minutes and strain out the herbs. Bottle. Apply with fingertips to chapped lips and skin.

Avoid exposure to sunlight when using St.-John's wort since it is phototoxic.

Bay Rum Lotion

bay rum
glycerin

Mix equal amounts of bay rum and glycerin. Use as a lotion for rough skin.

Athlete's Foot

Garlic for Athlete's Foot
  garlic clove

Split a clove of garlic. Rub it on the feet,
especially over and between the toes.
Apply twice a day. Try to let the feet stay
bare and dry several hours per day. For the
rest of the day, it's best to wear shoes that
"breathe" or have open work, like sandals.

Thyme Wash for Athlete's Foot
  ½ cup dried or 1 cup fresh thyme
  4 cups boiling water or apple-cider vinegar

To the boiling water, add fresh or dried
thyme. Cover and let steep for 10 minutes.
Pour into a small tub and soak the feet for
30 minutes. Dry without rinsing.

You can also steep thyme in apple-cider vinegar. Soak cotton balls in this tincture and rub over the foot and affected areas to kill the fungus.

Ringworm

Ringworm Relief Bath

½ cup lavender buds
½ cup peppermint
½ cup rosemary
1 cup Epsom salts (optional)

Make a bath bag of herbs to soak in the tub, using lavender buds, peppermint, and rosemary. Tie these up in a washcloth. You can use the bath bag up to three times before making a new one. Soak up to 20 minutes; dry completely. Peppermint and rosemary have antibacterial properties. Add Epsom salts, to bathwater, as desired.

Epsom-Salts Bath
   1 cup Epsom salts

Bathe daily for 2 weeks in an Epsom-salts bath, using 1 cup to bathwater.

❧

Ringworm Paste
   peppermint leaves or tea-tree essential oil
   1 to 2 drops water, as necessary

Crush peppermint leaves into a paste. Add 1 or 2 drops of water if necessary. Apply the paste to the fungal infection, rubbing into the area twice a day for 2 weeks or until the ringworm disappears.

   Apply tea-tree essential oil to the area the same way.

Impetigo & Fungal Infections

Impetigo Remedy
freshly hulled black walnuts and water

Boil the black walnuts in a little water. Make a compress and apply to the affected area.

Wash for Impetigo & Fungal Infections
¼ cup rosemary
¼ cup sage
1 teaspoon lemon juice
½ cup boiling water
½ cup honey

Add the rosemary and sage to the boiling water. Let steep for 15 minutes. Strain. Add lemon juice and stir in the honey. Apply to the affected areas twice a day.

DIGESTIVE UPSETS

Constipation

Here are teas, a juice, and other natural regulators that will help relieve constipation.

Flaxseed Tea
   1 heaping teaspoon psyllium seed or
   flaxseed
   1 cup boiling water

Make a tea by adding the psyllium seed or flaxseed to boiling water. Let steep for 10 minutes.

Prune Juice Remedy
   ⅔ cup prune juice

Drink a glass of prune juice before bed to help relieve constipation.

Senna-Leaf Tea

  3 senna leaves
  1 cup boiling water

Use senna leaves in boiling water to make
a tea. Steep for 10 minutes. For sluggish
bowels, the Amish favor senna-leaf tea.

Good Morning Regulator

  1 teaspoon lemon juice
  1 teaspoon olive oil
  1 teaspoon honey
  1 glass warm water

To keep you regular, every morning drink
lemon juice, olive oil, and honey in a glass
of warm water. Mix well.

Diarrhea

Blackberry juice, honey, and mullein help keep diarrhea in check.

Blackberry Juice

⅔ cup blackberry juice

Blackberry juice is wonderful for stopping diarrhea. Drink a glass of blackberry juice every 3 hours until you feel relief.

Honey Infusion

1 cup honey
1 teaspoon nutmeg
1 teaspoon allspice

Warm the honey and mix in the spices. Add 1 teaspoon or so of this to warm milk or tea. Drink every two hours until the diarrhea is reduced.

Mullein Diarrhea Relief

   1 teaspoon mullein leaves and flowers
   1 cup boiling water
   honey (optional)

Make a tea of mullein leaves and flowers.
Add 1 teaspoon to 1 cup boiling water.
Strain and add honey to taste. Or add the
honey infusion. (See above.)

Gastritis, Indigestion & Heartburn

Angelica Gas Relief

   angelica leaves, stems, and flowers
   vodka
   water or tea

Angelica, which has a licorice flavor, is
helpful for gastritis or excess gas. Use the
leaves, stems, and flowers. Place the herb
in a Mason jar. Cover with vodka. Let

steep for 2 weeks. Strain. Add a dropper of the tincture to your herb tea or just add to water and drink.

Herbal Substitutions: For the angelica, you can substitute basil, dill, or lovage. All these herbs are good digestives and help reduce flatulence.

Catnip & Peppermint Tea

dried peppermint
dried catnip
1 cup boiling water
honey (optional)

Mix equal amounts of dried peppermint and catnip. Use 1 teaspoon of this dried mixture in 1 cup boiling water. Strain and add honey to taste. Sip slowly when you have an upset stomach or indigestion.

Dill Flatulence & Colic Relief

4 medium potatoes
water
handful dill leaves and seeds

Peel the potatoes and cut them in chunks. Cover with water and a handful of dill leaves and seeds. Boil until soft. Set aside the potatoes and keep the water. Strain. Keep refrigerated.

For adults, give several tablespoons at a time. For babies, add 2 teaspoons to a bottle of formula. This remedy should keep for at least a week.

Chamomile Tummy Tincture

  chamomile flowers
  vodka

Place chamomile flowers in a jar and cover
with vodka. Let steep in a sunny window
for 2 weeks. Strain. Add more chamomile
flowers and steep again for 2 weeks. Strain
and bottle. Add a dropper of the tincture
to tea or juices for upset stomach. This
tincture will keep indefinitely.

Celery-Juice Tea Heartburn Relief

  celery stalks
  boiling water

Celery juice tea helps relieve heartburn.
Merely add some celery stalks to boiling
water and let simmer until soft. Strain and
sip the juice.

Lemonade Heartburn Relief

fresh lemons
honey or sugar
water

Drinking lemonade has been found to be
helpful for heartburn. Use fresh lemons.
Squeeze them and add sugar or honey
with water.

Oddly enough, lemon is great for acidic
disorders like arthritis and liver congestion.
It is also a carminative. Honey and lemon
is, of course, the standard treatment for a
sore throat.

Ulcers & Stomach Pain

Stomach Pain Remedy

1 tablespoon marsh mallow
1 tablespoon slippery-elm bark
1 tablespoon lobelia
1 tablespoon ginger root
2 cups water
1 tablespoon honey

Use equal amounts of marsh mallow, slippery-elm bark, lobelia, and ginger root. Place the herbs in a pan and cover them with water. Bring to a boil, reduce heat, cover, and simmer for 20 minutes. Strain. Add honey to the tea and mix well. Bottle, label, and refrigerate. This remedy will keep for about 6 months.

Take several teaspoons every 2 to 3 hours until stomach pains disappear.

Licorice Ulcer Relief

   dried licorice root
   olive oil
   1 tablespoon cod-liver oil

Make an infused oil of licorice root by placing the broken pieces of dried root in a jar and covering them with olive oil. Add 1 tablespoon cod-liver oil. Steep for 2 weeks.

   This concoction is very strong and numbing or relaxing when you feel pain. Take 1 teaspoon as needed every several hours. Do not exceed 4 teaspoons per day. This is also good for menstrual cramps.

   Licorice has been traditionally used for treating ulcers. It has antibacterial and mild antiviral effects; perhaps this is why it has worked so well.

Ulcer Tea

  licorice root powder
  slippery-elm root powder
  sage
  1 cup boiling water
  honey (optional)

Mix equal parts of licorice root powder, slippery-elm root powder, and sage. Store the herbal mixture in a sealed jar and label.

To use, add 1 teaspoon of the herbal mixture to boiling water. Steep for 15 minutes and strain. Add honey to taste.

Nausea & Motion Sickness

Peppermint Sniff

  peppermint extract or essential oil

Put several drops of peppermint extract or
essential oil onto a cotton ball to sniff to
get rid of nausea or motion sickness. You
can put this into a plastic bag and easily
carry it with you.

Spicy Stomach Plaster

  1 tablespoon ginger
  1 tablespoon cloves
  1 tablespoon cinnamon
  1 tablespoon black pepper
  1 tablespoon cayenne pepper
  blackstrap molasses

Mix the ginger, cloves, cinnamon, black
pepper, and cayenne pepper. Add enough

blackstrap molasses to make it the consistency of a stiff paste. Apply this to the stomach externally as a plaster.

Peppermint Tea

   1 tablespoon peppermint
   boiling water
   pinch ginger (optional)

Peppermint tea is wonderful for that sick feeling. You can also add a pinch of ginger to any this or any type of tea to help reduce nausea.

Or drink ginger ale; just make sure it contains real ginger.

TONICS

A tonic is an herbal drink used to boost the immune system and to give the body energy, vitality, and much-needed vitamins and minerals. Here are a few recipes you may want to try once a year. Drink the tonic up to three times a day for 1 week.

People used these tonics around springtime—when the rest of nature was renewing itself.

Blackberry Cordial

2 cups whole blackberries
¼ cup water
1½ cups sugar
⅛ teaspoon each nutmeg
⅛ teaspoon cinnamon
⅛ teaspoon ground cloves
3 cups brandy

Put blackberries in a pan with the water. Bring to boil, stirring constantly. Boil for 5 minutes. Strain out the seeds. Return the juice to the stove and add the sugar and spices. Bring to boil for another 5 minutes. Remove from heat and let cool to room temperature. Add the brandy. Seal in jars. Store in a dark cupboard. The cordial will be ready to use in 2 weeks.

Sip after dinner in a small cordial glass.

This tonic is good for getting the digestive juices flowing properly. Try it whenever you feel sluggish or bloated.

Rose-Hip Vitamin-C Booster

2 cups fresh rose hips
1½ cups water
juice of 1 lemon
3 cups sugar

Remove pips and finely chop or grind the rose hips. (Make sure you gather them from pesticide-free plants.) Set the rose hips aside. Pour the water into a pan and add the sugar and lemon juice. Bring the mixture to a boil and boil 5 minutes or until the sugar is dissolved.

Add the rose hips to the cooled sugar mixture. Mix completely. Pour the rose hip and sugar mixture into ice cube trays and freeze into cubes. To use, add a cube to juice, tea, or any cool drink.

This tonic will boost your immune system with vitamin C, an antioxidant.

Tonic Bitters

½ cup prickly-ash bark
½ cup poplar-root bark
2 tablespoons cinnamon sticks
1 tablespoon whole cloves
4 cups (1 quart or 1 liter) whiskey
4 cups (1 quart or 1 liter) apple cider

Smash barks and spices with a hammer. Put the prickly-ash bark, poplar-root bark, cinnamon sticks, whole cloves, whiskey, and apple cider in a jug. Let steep for 10 days. Strain and filter. Drink a wineglass of tonic after the evening meal.

This is a good all-around tonic. We've rounded off metric equivalents.

Violet Problem-Skin Tonic

   2 tablespoons dried Oregon grape root
   2 tablespoons licorice root
   ¼ cup fresh wild violet leaves and flowers
   4 cups boiling water

Add the dried Oregon grape root and
licorice root to boiling water. Let simmer
for 20 minutes. Then add the wild violet
and cover again. Let simmer on low for 10
more minutes. Strain, cool, bottle, and
refrigerate.

   Take 3 tablespoons per day for problem
skin. Use the same dosage for congestion,
sluggishness, arthritis, constipation, or
insomnia. The tonic acts as a blood
cleanser and a laxative.

Herbal Antiviral Tonic

½ gallon (1.9 liters) white wine
4 tablespoons sage leaves
4 tablespoons lavender buds
4 tablespoons thyme
4 tablespoons peppermint
4 tablespoons cloves
4 tablespoons garlic

Warm the white wine gently. Remove
from heat and add the sage, lavender buds,
thyme, peppermint, cloves, and garlic.
Cover and steep for 30 minutes. Strain.
Drink ½ cup two to three times a day.

This tonic cleanses and renews, getting
rid of almost any type of infection while
strengthening the immune system.

Rosemary & Ginseng "Cure-All" Tonic

½ gallon (1.9 liters) boiling water
⅛ cup powdered goldenseal root
¼ cup dried rosemary
¼ cup powdered ginseng root

Add the goldenseal root, rosemary, and ginseng root to boiling water. Reduce heat to simmer. Cover and let simmer for 30 minutes. Strain. Drink ½ cup twice a day.

This tonic benefits the body through the use of goldenseal. This herb was used in many patent medicines after the Civil War. It's also good for bacterial and fungal infections. Goldenseal also stimulates the liver function. Take it a half hour before meals.

Ginseng Tonic

½ cup chopped ginseng root
4 cups boiling water

Bring water to boiling. Reduce the heat, add the herb to the water, and cover. Simmer for 30 minutes. Strain, bottle. Drink ½ cup twice a day.

The Shakers were fond of the herb ginseng and used it in many of their tonics. Ginseng helps return body functions to normal. Be sure to use a good-quality ginseng root, whether fresh or dried.

Stinging Nettle Tonic

1 cup fresh stinging nettle
1 quart water
honey (optional)

When you pick fresh stinging nettle, be sure to use gloves. Bring the stinging nettle and water to a boil. Strain. Add honey to taste. Drink up to 3 cups of this tonic tea per day.

This tonic was well loved and passed down through the generations in Amish communities. Stinging nettle is high in necessary vitamins and nutrients.

Dandelion Spring Tonic

4 cups (1 quart or 0.9 liter) good wine
4 cups dandelion flowers with green parts
removed
1 tablespoon powdered dandelion root
1 cup honey
1 teaspoon cloves

Gently warm the wine. Add the dandelion
flowers, with all green parts removed; then
add the dandelion root, honey, and cloves.
Let the mixture steep in a closed container
for a week. Strain. Bottle and label. To use,
take 1 tablespoon before meals.

This dandelion spring tonic is a great
pick-me-up or energizer. It can also be
helpful for weight loss.

Sarsaparilla Tonic

¼ cup sarsaparilla
¼ cup spikenard root
¼ cup black birch bark
¼ cup yellow dock root
¼ cup spruce needles
2 cups boiling water (to cover herbs)
honey

Add the sarsaparilla, spikenard root, black birch bark, yellow dock root, and spruce needles to the boiling water. Maintain a hard boil for 20 minutes. Strain. Drink ½ cup, with honey added, twice a day.

Sarsaparilla tonic is very healing and good for digestion. It acts as a strong diuretic that helps dispel wastes and toxins. This tonic also promotes sweating.

Stomach Tonic

2 tablespoons dried snakeroot bark
2 tablespoons dried valerian root
2 tablespoons dried lavender buds
2 cups vodka

Put the snakeroot bark, valerian root, lavender buds, and the vodka in a Mason jar. Let steep in a sunny window for 2 weeks. Strain.

To calm a jittery, nervous stomach and aid digestion, take this tonic. It is also helpful for relaxation and sleep and for headache relief. Take 1 teaspoon before bedtime.

ARTHRITIS, GOUT & MUSCLE ACHES

Many believe that arthritis can be caused by allergens, such as those found in plants in the nightshade family, Solanaceae—tomatoes, white potatoes, eggplant, zucchini, and peppers. In these cases, it's merely a matter of avoiding suspected allergens and toxins or not eating specified foods. One can relieve arthritis and gout with a few remedies that help allay the pain while detoxifying the system.

Others have proposed that arthritis is caused by mineral imbalances in the diet and, therefore, in the body. Also, some have found relief from arthritislike symptoms from eating foods rich in antioxidants or taking antioxidant supplements.

Muscle aches usually come from overexertion. Pain relievers and rest are usually all that you need in most cases. A diet rich in fruits and vegetables as well as necessary minerals helps prevent muscle cramps.

❧
Toxin Flushes

Fresh Carrot Juice Toxin Flush: Fast for 3 days, drinking nothing but pure water and up to 3 glasses of fresh carrot juice a day.

Grape Juice Toxin Flush: Drink 3 glasses a day of pure Concord grape juice (no sugar added) instead of the carrot juice. Complete this fasting regimen in 3 days.

Aloe-Vera Toxin Flush: Drink just 3 fluid ounces (⅜ cup) of aloe-vera juice with 1 teaspoon of olive oil in it once a day during a three-day fast.

Green-Tea Salad Dressing

2 teaspoons diced garlic
3 tablespoons olive oil
5 tablespoons clover honey
¼ cup green tea
1 tablespoon apple-cider vinegar
½ teaspoon cayenne pepper (optional)

Sauté the garlic in the oil and set aside. Mix the clover honey, green tea, apple-cider vinegar, and cayenne pepper. Simmer the honey mixture for 5 minutes and strain. Add the garlic oil mixture and blend. Pour the salad dressing into a sealed container and refrigerate. Shake to mix. Use 1 to 2 tablespoons on your salad per day.

This traditional salad dressing for relief of arthritis pain can be used every day. If you are allergic to foods in the nightshade family, omit the cayenne pepper.

Willow Joint-Pain Liniment

4 cups rubbing alcohol
1 cup dried willow bark
½ cup dried rosemary
½ cup lemon peel

Mix the alcohol with the herbs and lemon peel. Place the mixture in a sunny window for 2 weeks. Shake daily. Strain. Use this liniment to rub on joints and surrounding areas. This liniment helps relieve arthritis and gout pain and inflammation.

Wintergreen Steam Inhalation

handful wintergreen
boiling water

Put a handful of wintergreen plant in a bowl of boiling water. Cover your head with a towel and drape it over the bowl so that you can inhale the vapors. Inhale deeply. Wintergreen is a traditional remedy that helps ease arthritis and other pain.

❦

Elderberry Arthritis Remedy

  2 cups boiling water
  ½ cup elderberries
  ¼ cup dried white yarrow leaves and
    flowers
  1 cup honey

Add the elderberries and white yarrow to the boiling water. Cover and steep for 20 minutes. Strain. Add honey and mix well.

Sip ½ cup every 6 to 8 hours until pain subsides. Do not drink more than 2 cups per day.

Pokeberry Tea

dried pokeberry
1 cup boiling water

To the boiling water, add a dried pokeberry. Drink one cup a day.

The Blackfoot tribe passed this remedy
onto American pioneers to help prevent
and ease the pain of arthritis.

Peanut Oil Rubs

2 cups peanut oil
1 cup lavender buds

Warm the peanut oil gently, then add the
lavender. Place in a jar and let soak for 1
week. Strain. Once a week after a bath,
massage the oil well into the skin all over
the body.

Edgar Cayce, the American psychic and healer, recommends peanut-oil rubs for soothing arthritis. I've added the herb lavender for extra healing benefits.

Arthritis-Easing Rosemary Bath

1 cup Epsom salts
½ cup dried rosemary

Every day for a month try this. Pour the Epsom salts into hot bathwater. Tie up the dried rosemary into a washcloth and let it soak in the bathwater. Soak in the tub for 20 minutes in the evening before bed.

Arthritis Toddy

2 tablespoons olive oil
1 cup warm milk

Add olive oil to warm milk before bedtime. The oil reportedly reduces inflammation.

Poultice for Arthritis & Tendonitis
comfrey, epazote, or mullein leaves

Dip the leaves of comfrey, epazote, or mullein into hot water. Place the warmed leaves on the affected area as a hot poultice. The poultice should not be hot enough to burn. Leave on for 15 minutes; replace with new warmed leaves.

Epazote (*Teloxys ambrosioides*) is also called worm seed or Mexican tea.

Cool Comfrey Compress for Sprains
1 cup chopped comfrey leaf
½ cup chamomile flowers
½ cup marjoram leaves
4 cups boiling water

Add the chopped fresh comfrey leaf, chamomile flowers, and marjoram leaves to boiling water. Let cool and strain. Add ice to the herbal water. Dip a cloth into the cool herbal water and apply it to the sprain for 30 minutes, dipping frequently.

❧

Soothing Lavender & Peppermint Soak

  2 cups boiling water
  ½ cup lavender buds
  ½ cup peppermint leaves
  1 cup Epsom salts or ½ cup baking soda

In boiling water, add the lavender buds and peppermint leaves to make a tea. Strain. Add the herbal tea to warm bath-water with Epsom salts or baking soda.

  Take a warm herbal soak in a tub when you feel overworked and your muscles and everything ache. It will help you feel ener-gized and relieve the pain.

Soothing Thyme & Eucalyptus Soak

  2 tablespoons dry mustard
  2 tablespoons thyme
  2 tablespoons eucalyptus leaves

Tie up a washcloth or muslin bag with dry
mustard, thyme, and eucalyptus leaves. Tie
tightly and let the bag float in a tub of
warm water. Squeeze over the body frequently and soak up to 20 minutes.

Massage Oil for Muscle Aches

  ¼ cup hyssop
  ¼ cup lavender
  ¼ cup marjoram
  2 cups peanut oil

Let the hyssop, lavender, and marjoram
steep in the peanut oil for 2 weeks in a
sunny window. Strain. Massage into tired,
overworked muscles.

Soothing Witch-Hazel Rub

1 cup witch hazel
peppermint leaves
2 tablespoons lanolin
1 cup peanut oil

To the witch hazel, add as many peppermint leaves as you can. Let them soak 1 week. Strain. Add liquid lanolin and peanut oil. Mix well. Kept in the refrigerator, this will be a thick lotion.

Use this lotion as a rub for aching joints and muscles.

HEADACHES

Almost everyone gets headaches. Most of the time, headaches result from plain old stress. But there are other causes too, like sinusitis, allergies, caffeine (too much or too little a daily dose), or overindulgence in alcohol. Or you may be prone to migraines. Here are some remedies sure to ease the pounding pain and pressure of any type of headache you may suffer.

A serious headache in someone who normally does not suffer headaches could be a sign of a serious problem, like an embolism or blood clot on the brain. Seek medical care promptly.

If you suffer from allergies, you may notice along with headaches a stuffy nose, runny eyes, sneezing, and even changes in temperament. Honey has been used for centuries to help ease allergies. Honey slowly works at getting rid of symptoms, and eventually the allergies disappear. Use honey harvested in your own region if you want to reduce your susceptibility to local pollens. Herbalists have speculated that the microparticles of pollen in honey may help the same way allergy shots do.

The Honey Cure: Traditionally, people with allergies took 1 tablespoon of honey after each meal. Or they added 1 tablespoon of honey to 1 cup of warm water and drank it at bedtime. You can also chew honeycomb to keep the sinuses open and dry, since this also helps with headaches. Or make a hot drink with the honeycomb.

Honey Milk for Headaches

   1 cup milk
   1 tablespoon honey
   dash lemon juice

Heat the milk gently; stir in the honey and
lemon juice, and sip before sleep.

Juniper & Rosemary Temple Rub

   2 tablespoons rubbing alcohol
   10 drops juniper essential oil
   10 drops rosemary essential oil

Add the alcohol, juniper essential oil, and
rosemary essential oil to a bottle. Cap and
shake the bottle to mix. Apply this mixture
to fingertips and rub into the temples and
surrounding areas to help ease pain.

   Substitutions: You can use 10 drops
lavender essential oil and 10 drops pepper-

mint essential oil in place of the rosemary and juniper essential oils.

This is a good all-around headache remedy, but it is also good for hangover headaches.

Paper-Bag Plaster

brown paper bag
1 cup boiling water
¼ cup dried lavender
¼ cup dried peppermint
ice water

Tear a brown paper bag (sack) into strips the size of the forehead. Next you'll need a bowl of cool water; add some ice cubes if you wish. To the boiling water, add the lavender and peppermint. Cover and let steep. Strain. Add the herbal water to the ice water.

Place the brown paper in the ice water and then plaster it to the forehead. Lie down. As the paper dries, dip into the water again and once more plaster it to the head. Do this for at least 25 minutes or until the headache eases.

Mustard Foot Bath

hot water
2 teaspoons powdered mustard

Since a hot foot bath diverts the blood supply from the head to the foot area, it helps ease headaches.

To a small foot tub, add hot water—as hot as you can stand. Mix the powdered mustard into the water, and soak your feet for 15 to 20 minutes.

Apple-Cider-Vinegar Cold Compress

cool water
apple-cider vinegar

A cold compress is good for sinus headaches. Use equal amounts of cool water and apple-cider vinegar. Wring a cloth in this and apply it to the forehead.

Cold Compress for Sinus Congestion

boiling water
dried thyme or dried eucalyptus
dried basil

For sinus congestion, boil some water and add equal amounts of dried thyme or eucalyptus, and basil. You can inhale the steam.

Or let the mixture cool, add ice, and use a cloth, wrung out, to apply it on closed eyes and press it around the nose and forehead.

White-Willow Tincture

½ gallon (2 liters) vodka
1 pound (500 g) white-willow leaves

Put the vodka and white-willow leaves in a closed jar and let the jar sit in a sunny window for 2 weeks. Shake daily. Strain and bottle. Use 1 dropper of the white-willow tincture for headaches.

White willow was often used by Native Americans to relieve pain. From white willow we have isolated essential ingredients for modern-day aspirin. This tincture is good for feverish headaches.

Herbal Soak for Menstrual Headaches

½ cup sweet marjoram
½ cup Roman chamomile
½ cup lavender

Wrap the sweet marjoram, Roman chamomile, and lavender in a muslin cloth and tie tightly. Toss this herbal bag into a warm tub and soak in the tub for 20 to 25 minutes.

Use this remedy at that time of the month when you feel irritated, bloated, and headachy.

Feverfew Migraine Remedy

large leaf or 1 teaspoon dried feverfew
2 cups boiling water (for tea)

Eat 1 large leaf of feverfew daily to prevent migraine headaches. If fresh feverfew is unavailable, add 1 teaspoon of the dried herb to 2 cups of boiling water and drink no more than 1 cup of this tea daily.

This easy remedy is specific for migraines, but don't overdose on this herb. Use no more than this recommended dose.

Headache Tea Blend

  1 tablespoon skullcap
  2 tablespoons rose petals
  1 tablespoon sweet marjoram
  4 cups boiling water
  ½ cup brown sugar or to taste

Add the skullcap, rose petals, and marjoram to boiling water. Remove from heat, cover, and steep for 15 minutes. Strain. Dissolve the brown sugar in the tea, adding the amount you prefer to taste. Cool and bottle.

Refrigerate and keep this headache tea blend on hand. Drink a glass of the tea up to three times per day for a headache.

This blend is especially good for stress and grief headaches.

❦

Lavender Headache Tea

1 teaspoon dried or 3 teaspoons fresh lavender buds
1 cup boiling water

Pour boiling water over the lavender buds. Cover and steep for 5 minutes. Sweeten to taste. Drink up to 2 cups.

This pleasant tea is very relaxing and helpful for migraines and other pounding headaches.

Valerian & Licorice Headache Tea

 1 cup boiling water
 2 teaspoons valerian root
 1 teaspoon licorice root

Add the valerian and licorice roots to the boiling water. Again, bring the water and herbs to a boil and simmer 10 minutes. Strain and drink. The licorice adds sweetness and helps mask the awful taste of the valerian.

 This is especially relaxing and good for stress or anxiety. Since valerian acts as a sedative, only drink this in the evening or when you are not driving or operating machinery.

Peppermint Headache Tea

⅜ cup dried peppermint
4 cups boiling water

Pour the boiling water over the dried peppermint. Cover and steep for 10 minutes. Strain. Put the peppermint herb tea in the refrigerator. Drink ½ cup up to 2 cups to rid yourself of a headache or nausea.

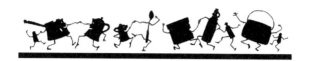

Part 2
BEAUTY & LUXURY

In this part, you'll find recipes to make your own perfumes, sweet waters, colognes, and aftershaves. You'll also discover skin lotions, creams, lip balms, and lip gloss. Helpful treatments for acne, scars, and stretch marks may "save your skin."

For hair care, you'll discover shampoos, conditioners, rinses, gels, dressings, and colorants for all types of hair. You'll be able to create facial scrubs, masks, toners, and astringents, following traditional Victorian recipes.

For the bath, you'll find bath oils, herbal infusions, foams, bubbles, salts, scented bags, and after-bath dusting powders.

To help you sleep, you'll find traditional sleep potions, including teas, salves, an onion sandwich, and dream pillows. Also, learn gentle ways to quiet children and ready them for sleep.

Natural beauty products are easy to create and results are often amazing. It only takes a few moments to mix up a recipe, but this pampering can renew the soul and wonderfully enhance the appearance in lasting ways.

PERFUMES, COLOGNES, SWEET WATERS & AFTERSHAVES

Women's Perfumes & Colognes

Once you master the basic recipe, perfumes and colognes are quite easy to create. You'll be excited when you begin to experiment with the many possible scent combinations. Here are a few favorite time-honored scents.

Tender Rose Perfume

¼ cup vodka
60 drops rose essential oil
16 drops sandalwood essential oil
10 drops lemon essential oil
¼ teaspoon jojoba oil (fixative)

Pour the vodka, rose essential oil, sandalwood essential oil, lemon essential oil, and jojoba oil into a perfume bottle. Shake well and allow the solution to sit about a week before use. Although this perfume is expensive to make, the smell is exquisite.

If you prefer, you can substitute vitamin E oil for the jojoba oil, and shake the perfume before each use. Jojoba oil is alcohol-soluble and acts as a fixative.

Spicy Girl
¼ cup (2 fluid ounces or 60 ml) vodka
1 tablespoon glycerin
8 drops cinnamon essential oil
10 drops clove essential oil
20 drops bergamot essential oil

Blend the vodka and glycerin with the cinnamon, clove, and bergamot essential oils. Pour the mixture into a tightly closed container. Allow the scents to meld together several days before use.

Sweet Eden Perfume

¼ cup jojoba oil
½ teaspoon pure vanilla extract
20 drops jasmine essential oil
18 drops tuberose essential oil
10 drops sweet orange essential oil
10 drops rose essential oil
10 drops mimosa essential oil
8 drops bergamot essential oil
8 drops musk

Blend the jojoba oil, musk, and vanilla extract with the jasmine, tuberose, sweet orange, rose, mimosa, and bergamot essential oils. Let the mixture sit about 4 days in a closed container and bottle.

This recipe, found in an old apothecary's notebook, created gallons of perfume to bottle and sell. Since some original ingredients are now unavailable, I've modified the recipe slightly and cut it down to size.

Warm Charm

½ cup vodka
½ teaspoon jojoba oil (fixative)
25 drops lavender essential oil
20 drops rosemary essential oil
15 drops lemon essential oil
15 drops clove essential oil
15 drops geranium essential oil
10 drops neroli essential oil

Blend the vodka, jojoba oil, and the lavender, rosemary, lemon, clove, geranium, and neroli essential oils well. Let the mixture steep for 1 week in a closed container before use. Bottle.

Morning Dawn

2 tablespoons jojoba oil or almond oil
12 drops ylang-ylang essential oil
6 drops clary-sage essential oil
4 drops vetiver essential oil
2 drops lavender essential oil

Blend the jojoba oil and the ylang-ylang, clary-sage, vetiver, and lavender essential oils. Bottle. Shake well every day. Let steep for 3 days before using.

Cupid's Dream

 ¼ cup vodka
 1 tablespoon glycerin
 20 drops ylang-ylang essential oil
 18 drops mandarin essential oil
 12 drops neroli essential oil

Mix the vodka, glycerin, and the ylang-ylang, mandarin, and neroli essential oils well. Let the mixture steep for 1 to 2 weeks in a closed container. Bottle.

Sweet Waters

Sweet waters were used to freshen up between baths, which had been less frequent than today's routine daily shower. Toilet waters and toilet vinegars also helped to refresh people on hot, dusty days before the advent of air conditioning. Usually these sweet waters were splashed on from a wash basin or used to refresh the body by soaking a handkerchief with them and daubing them on pulse points.

The fresh and light scent of these waters is weaker than that of traditional home-made perfumes. If you wish, you can use the same scents as those of your perfume. That way, the scents will complement each other, and you can layer them. Today, we use the sweet waters in much the same way; we simply call them body splashes. The first two recipes are old-fashioned standbys.

Note: If you're buying distilled water or vinegar, 5 fluid ounces (150 ml) equals ⅝ cup.

Rosewater

  ¾ cup distilled water
  ¼ cup dried rose petals
  6 drops rose essential oil

In a jar, add the rose petals to the distilled water and close the lid tightly. Shake the jar to make sure that the petals are covered with water. Set the jar in a sunny window for 2 to 3 days. Strain. Add rose essential oil drops and place the mixture in an atomizer spray bottle or pretty jar.

Keep refrigerated for a cool, soothing spritz. Rosewater is relaxing and good for the skin.

Lavender Sweet Vinegar

⅝ cup good wine vinegar
¼ cup dried lavender buds
18 drops lavender essential oil

Put lavender buds in a jar with the wine vinegar. Close the lid on the jar. Set the mixture in a sunny window for 2 to 3 days. Strain and add the lavender essential oil. Shake well and bottle.

Use lavender sweet vinegar on days when you want to relieve stress or a headache. Spritz or splash it on the skin.

Jasmine Sweet Water

20 drops jasmine essential oil
⅝ cup distilled water
4 drops jojoba oil (fixative)

Add the jasmine essential oil to the water.
Add a few drops of jojoba oil, which acts
as a fixative. Mix well. Spritz or splash on
before a big night out on the town.

Chamomile Sweet Water

¾ cup distilled water
¼ cup chamomile tea
20 drops chamomile essential oil

Make strong chamomile tea using a tea
bag or 1 tablespoon chamomile to ¼ cup
boiling water. Steep 10 minutes. Add ¾
cup distilled water and chamomile essential oil. For a refreshing applelike scent,
splash this sweet water on your skin.

Peppermint Sweet Vinegar

¾ cup good wine vinegar
½ cup peppermint tea
12 drops peppermint essential oil

Make a strong peppermint tea with 1 tablespoon peppermint or 1 tea bag and ½ cup boiling water. Steep 10 minutes. Blend the vinegar, peppermint tea, and peppermint essential oil.

This is a refreshing splash that helps wake you up and boost energy. It also helps you cool down when you're hot and sweaty.

Sweet-Woodruff Water

¾ cup distilled water
¼ cup sweet woodruff tea
20 drops sweet woodruff essential oil

Make a strong tea with 1 tablespoon or 1 tea bag of sweet woodruff to ¼ cup boiling water. Steep 10 minutes. Blend the distilled water, sweet woodruff tea, and sweet woodruff essential oil well. Sweet woodruff has a pleasing cherry-vanilla scent. Splash on this sweet water.

Sandalwood & Orange Sweet Water

orange peel from 1 orange
⅝ cup distilled water
15 drops sandalwood essential oil
6 drops sweet orange essential oil

Add orange peel to the boiling water. Remove from heat and cool. Strain. Add the sandalwood and sweet orange essential oils and mix well. Let sit for several days.

Spritz the sweet water on the body to help clear the mind and dispel dark moods.

Men's Colognes

Men's colognes are easy to create. Instead of floral scents, which are more suitable for women, use earthy, woody scents with a touch of spice.

Gentleman's Cologne

⅝ cup (5 fluid ounces or 150 ml) vodka
2 tablespoons distilled water
15 drops lavender essential oil
8 drops thyme essential oil
6 drops lemongrass essential oil
cinnamon stick

Mix the vodka, the distilled water, and the lavender, thyme, and lemongrass essential oils. Add the cinnamon stick and cover. Let steep for 2 weeks. Remove the cinnamon stick. This is an old favorite.

Woodsman

¾ cup vodka
1 tablespoon or 1 tea bag rosemary
½ cup boiling water
15 drops sandalwood essential oil
8 drops coriander essential oil
¼ teaspoon jojoba oil

Make strong rosemary tea with dried rosemary or the tea bag and the boiling water. Let steep for 10 minutes. Blend the vodka, rosemary tea, sandalwood essential oil, coriander essential oil, and jojoba oil well. Let the mixture sit for about 1 week tightly covered.

Macho Man

   2 cups (1 pint or 480 ml) dark rum
   ½ cup bay leaves
   2 tablespoons whole cloves
   2 cinnamon sticks
   6 to 8 drops bay essential oil

Mix the rum, bay leaves, cloves, cinnamon sticks, and bay essential oil. Seal the mixture in a jar. Let it steep for 2 weeks. Strain, bottle, and label.

Mysterious Man

   ⅜ cup vodka
   2 tablespoons distilled water
   8 drops frankincense essential oil
   6 drops clary-sage essential oil

Blend the vodka, distilled water, and the frankincense and clary-sage essential oils well. Seal and let sit for 2 to 3 days. Bottle.

Daredevil
  ½ cup vodka
  2 tablespoons distilled water
  8 drops vetiver essential oil
  6 drops basil essential oil
  6 drops pine essential oil

Blend the vodka, distilled water, and the vetiver, basil, and pine essential oils. Steep in a tightly closed container for 1 week.

Apply when you're in a rakish mood.

Men's Aftershaves

Refreshing Aftershave

  2 cups distilled water
  1 cup witch hazel
  2 tablespoons tincture of benzoin
  10 drops lime essential oil
  8 drops bergamot essential oil

Mix the distilled water, witch hazel, benzoin, lime essential oil, and bergamot essential oil well. Seal in a jar. Let sit for several days. Splash on the face after shaving to close the pores and tone the skin.

Teddy Bear Aftershave

  2 teaspoons lavender buds
  ¾ cup boiling water
  1 cup dark rum
  10 drops rosemary essential oil
  8 drops peppermint essential oil

Make lavender tea, using lavender buds and the boiling water. Steep for 10 minutes. Cool and strain. Add the dark rum, rosemary essential oil, and peppermint essential oil. Bottle. Let the mixture sit for about 1 week before using it.

Piney Aftershave

¼ cup witch hazel
1 cup vodka
4 cups distilled water
2 tablespoons glycerin
½ teaspoon juniper essential oil

Blend the witch hazel, vodka, distilled water, glycerin, and juniper essential oil well. Bottle. Let the mixture sit for several days before usage.

SKIN CARE

Soothing Lotions & Creams

Rose Cream
   4 tablespoons rosewater (rose-petal tea)
   2 tablespoons melted beeswax
   6 tablespoons sweet almond oil
   6 drops vitamin E oil
   4 to 6 drops rose essential oil (optional)

Use 2 tablespoons of rose petals to make a strong tea or rosewater in ½ cup boiling water. Let steep for 10 minutes and set aside. Melt the beeswax in the top of a double boiler. Blend in the sweet almond oil and vitamin E oil. Remove from heat, and stirring constantly, add the rosewater and rose essential oil. Beat vigorously until cooled and the mixture is fluffy and whitened.

For a more concentrated scent, add rose essential oil. The rose, because of its cleansing, astringent properties and its benefits to skin, has been used for centuries in beauty products.

Rose cream is a good facial moisturizer and cleansing cream for removing makeup. Place the cream in a pretty jar and keep plenty on hand to smooth rough skin, day or night.

Lavender Face Cream

¾ cup olive oil
¼ cup liquid lanolin
1 tablespoon grated beeswax
⅔ cup lavender sweet water
⅓ cup glycerin
25 drops lavender essential oil
25 drops tea-tree essential oil

Warm the olive oil and lanolin in a small saucepan. Add grated beeswax and stir until the beeswax is melted. Remove from heat and cool. Blend glycerin and lavender water in a blender. Add the oil mixture in a small stream with the blender at high speed. When the mixture is thick, add the lavender essential oil (healing) and the tea-tree (antibacterial) essential oil.

Cold Cream Makeup Remover

1 cup sweet almond oil
4 tablespoons melted beeswax
½ cup rosewater
1 tablespoon powdered borax
7 drops rose essential oil

Melt the beeswax with the sweet almond oil and dissolve the borax in the rosewater. Add the rosewater and borax mixture to the oil slowly, and stir constantly until cool. Then add the rose essential oil. Pour into jars.

Aloe-Vera Face & Body Cream

¾ cup sweet almond oil
¼ cup liquid lanolin
1 tablespoon grated beeswax
⅔ cup lavender sweet water
⅓ cup aloe-vera gel
15 drops chamomile essential oil
12 drops lavender essential oil
2 capsules or ¼ teaspoon vitamin E oil

Melt the sweet almond oil, lanolin, and beeswax in a heat-resistant ceramic or glass saucepan over low heat. Cool to room temperature. Add the lavender sweet water, aloe-vera gel, chamomile essential oil, lavender essential oil, and vitamin E oil. Whip them in a blender until creamy. Store the cream in a covered jar.

Chamomile Dry-Skin Lotion

½ cup olive oil
¼ cup chamomile flowers

Soak the chamomile flowers in the olive oil for 1 to 2 weeks. Strain. Apply the skin lotion all over the body and massage in well.

This can serve as a good massage oil for dehydrated skin. It heals wounds and cuts, and it's also good for psoriasis.

No-Wrinkle Lotion

2 tablespoons basil tea leaves
2 tablespoons linden flower or lemon-balm tea
2 tablespoons jojoba oil
2 teaspoons honey

Use ½ cup boiling water to 1 tablespoon basil to make a strong basil tea. Mix 1 tablespoon linden flower or lemon balm to ½ cup boiling water to make linden flower or lemon balm tea. Steep teas for 10 minutes and set aside. You will only be using 2 tablespoons each of these brewed teas.

Mix the basil tea, linden flower tea, jojoba oil, and honey well. Apply the lotion to clean skin. Before bedtime, smooth it on the face or just under the eyes.

Basic Hand Lotion

2 tablespoons quince seeds
2 cups boiling distilled water
½ cup glycerin
½ cup alcohol

Pour the boiling water onto the quince seeds. Soak them overnight. Strain, add the glycerin and alcohol, mix well, and bottle. Use this hand lotion to soften skin.

Rich & Creamy Lotion

1 tablespoon unflavored gelatin
1 cup water
1 tablespoon jojoba oil
2 teaspoons cod-liver oil
6 to 8 drops red food coloring (optional)

Dissolve 1 tablespoon unflavored gelatin in ¼ cup cold water. Add ¾ cup boiling water to this and let cool. Add ½ cup of the gelatin mixture to the jojoba oil and cod-liver oil while running the blender. Pour in a small stream.

If you wish to give the cream a pretty pink tint, you can color it. When the mixture is creamy, add several drops of red food coloring and blend.

Rosewater & Glycerin Hand Lotion

  2 tablespoons rosewater
  30 drops glycerin
  1 teaspoon sweet almond oil

Mix the rosewater, glycerin, and sweet
almond oil well, beating by hand with a
wooden spoon or whisk.

  This traditional hand lotion is good for
aging skin. If you like it, double or triple
the recipe.

Oatmeal Dry-Skin Lotion

1½ cups distilled water
½ cup instant rolled oats
¼ to ½ cup grated beeswax
15 drops lavender, rose, jasmine, or rose
  geranium essential oil

Bring water to a boil. Remove from heat, add the rolled oats, and strain. Return water to heat, add the beeswax, and gently heat until melted. Cool to room temperature, beating well, and adding the essential oil. Store the skin lotion in a plastic bag or glass jar.

Apply to dry skin.

Simple Lotion

1 cup jojoba oil or olive oil
1 tablespoon melted beeswax
1 tablespoon lecithin
½ teaspoon vitamin E oil
2 cups ice-cold distilled water

Melt the jojoba oil, beeswax, lecithin, and vitamin E oil on low heat. Pour the ice-cold water into a blender or into a bowl if you use a hand mixer. Slowly add melted jojoba or olive oil, beeswax, lecithin, and vitamin E oil in a stream to the water as you blend on low speed. The mixture will soon turn creamy.

You can add essential oils if you want a scented lotion. This skin lotion keeps well. It is easily absorbed into the skin, especially if you use jojoba or olive oil. You may use another oil if you wish.

Acne, Scars & Stretch Marks

Avoid using oils on burns; aloe vera is best for cooling and healing burns. Silky Skin Cream and zinc with vitamin E work well to fade and prevent scars and stretch marks.

❧

Zinc & Vitamin E Treatment

  zinc oxide
  vitamin E oil

Apply both vitamin E oil and zinc oxide to a cut or wound to help prevent scarring as it begins to heal.

  A good hand lotion may aid absorption. Zinc oxide is a mild antiseptic that's great for skin.

Silky Skin Cream

3 tablespoons jojoba oil
1 tablespoon peanut oil
1¼ teaspoons grated beeswax
20 drops lavender essential oil
4 drops frankincense essential oil

Melt the jojoba oil, peanut oil, and beeswax together over low heat. Remove them from heat and let cool. Add the lavender and frankincense essential oils.

Pour the mixture into a small container. Massage the cream into the skin daily to help fade and prevent stretch marks and scars.

Acne-Healing Face Cream

3 tablespoons jojoba oil or cold-pressed,
   cold-processed castor oil
1¼ tablespoons olive oil
¼ teaspoon lanolin
½ teaspoon grated beeswax
3 tablespoons rosewater
1 tablespoon aloe-vera gel
1 teaspoon glycerin
10 drops tea-tree essential oil

Melt the jojoba or castor oil, olive oil,
lanolin, and beeswax over low heat. Cool
them to room temperature. The rosewater
should be the same temperature as the oils.
Beat the oils with a mixer, while pouring
the rosewater into the bowl in a steady
stream. It will turn thick and very creamy.
Place the cream in a pretty, decorative jar.
You can use this cream as a night cream to
help skin stay smooth and clear. It's also
soothing for chapped and cracked skin.

Lip Balms & Lip Gloss

Orange Lip Balm

½ teaspoon melted beeswax
½ teaspoon melted cocoa butter
1 teaspoon olive oil
2 drops sweet orange essential oil
1 capsule or ⅛ teaspoon vitamin E oil
½ teaspoon honey

Melt the beeswax and cocoa butter gently. Mix the olive oil, sweet orange essential oil, and vitamin E oil. Add the beeswax, cocoa butter, honey, and mix well. Pour the mixture into little containers and stir until the mixture begins to harden.

Use as you would any lip balm. This one is sweet and tasty.

Kissing-Sweet Lip Balm

½ cup sweet almond oil
1 capsule or ⅛ teaspoon vitamin E oil
2 tablespoons melted beeswax
¾ teaspoon cherry, peppermint, coconut, or
   vanilla flavoring

Gently warm the sweet almond oil, vita-min E oil, and beeswax together until the beeswax melts. Then you can add ¾ tea-spoon of any flavoring you wish—cherry, peppermint, coconut, or vanilla. Mix well.

Let cool to find out how hard the gloss is. If it is too creamy, add a little more beeswax and reheat. If it is too hard, add a little more oil. When you've gotten the right consistency, pour the mixture into little jars or lip-gloss containers.

This makes a great gift for teens or people who love the outdoors or have chapped lips.

Sheer & Easy Lip Gloss

1 teaspoon petroleum jelly
2 teaspoons aloe-vera gel
6 to 8 drops vanilla, cherry, or raspberry flavoring
leftover lipstick, any shade

Mix the petroleum jelly, aloe-vera gel, flavoring, and a small amount of lipstick well to make this sheer lip color.

You can place the lip gloss in tiny containers, such as pill dispensers. Make several different shades for each compartment. Experiment.

HAIR CARE

Shampoos

Save old shampoo bottles for these homemade shampoos. Don't forget to label the
bottle(s).

Gentle Aloe-Vera Shampoo
  ¾ cup castile soap flakes
  4 cups boiling water
  5 tablespoons lavender buds
  1 cup aloe-vera gel

Pour the boiling water over the lavender
buds and castile soap flakes. Let the mixture steep until cool. Mix in the aloe-vera
gel. This recipe makes more than 1 quart
(about 1 liter) of shampoo.

You can substitute another herb for the

lavender. To bring out natural highlights, brunettes could add sage or rosemary. Blondes could add chamomile or calendula. For oily hair, try thyme or lemongrass. For dry hair, try chamomile or lavender.

Soapwort Shampoo

  2 cups soapwort
  2 cups boiling water
  2 cups strong herbal tea

Pour the boiling water over the soapwort. Cover and let steep until cool. Strain. Mix with the herbal tea and seal the liquid in a bottle. Let this mixture sit a day or more before using.

  This is a mild shampoo made from the naturally sudsy soapwort. It doesn't lather up like commercial shampoos, but it does cleanse quite well. Shake before use or try

adding some glycerin to keep the shampoo
well mixed.

Herbs recommended for the strong
herbal tea are nettle, spearmint, rosemary,
thyme, or fennel. Use about 2 tablespoons
dried herb or 4 tea bags to 2 cups boiling
water. Let steep for 10 minutes.

Honey Shampoo

    1 cup mild liquid soap or baby shampoo
    2 cups strong herbal tea
    1 cup honey

Mix the liquid soap, herbal tea, and honey.
Pour the mixture into a bottle. Shake well
before using. This shampoo is especially
good for dry hair and for healing the scalp.
This makes about 1 pint or 500 ml of
shampoo. Rose-petal tea works well in this
recipe.

Herbal Shampoo

1 cup distilled water
2 teaspoons dried or 1 tablespoon fresh rosemary
½ cup mild liquid soap or baby shampoo
½ cup glycerin
¼ cup borax powder

Bring water to boil, add the rosemary, and let steep until water has cooled to room temperature. Strain. Add the liquid soap, glycerin, and borax powder. Blend. The mixture will thicken overnight. This recipe makes about 2 cups (1 pint or 500 ml) of shampoo.

Shampoo as you normally would. Save an old shampoo bottle for this homemade version. Don't forget to label it.

Homemade Dandruff Shampoo

1 cup mild liquid soap or baby shampoo
¼ cup willow-bark tea
35 drops lavender essential oil
18 drops rosemary essential oil
10 drops cedarwood essential oil

To make the willow-bark tea, pour 1 cup of water over a handful of willow leaves, steep until cool, and strain. Mix the liquid soap, willow-bark tea, and essential oils well. Pour the shampoo into a squeeze bottle.

Use a small amount every other day as a shampoo. Massage 3 to 5 minutes into the scalp and rinse very well. This will help control dandruff.

Conditioners & Rinses

Hot-Oil Conditioner

¼ cup dried rosemary
1 cup olive oil

Heat the olive oil gently until well warmed. Place the rosemary in the olive oil. Seal the mixture and set it aside for 2 to 3 days. Strain. Bottle the hot-oil hair conditioner.

Now, whenever you want a hot-oil treatment, warm 1 tablespoon of the oil conditioner in a microwave-safe bowl. Rub between your fingers and massage the conditioner into your scalp and hair. Wrap your head in a towel and allow 30 minutes for it to soak in. Shampoo as usual. This hot-oil conditioner is good for dry hair. It also appears to help stimulate hair growth.

Coconut Oil Conditioner

½ cup coconut oil
8 drops lavender essential oil
4 drops sandalwood essential oil

Warm the coconut oil since it is solid at room temperature, although it melts at body temperature. Remove from heat, cool slightly, and add the essential oils, mixing well. Pour into a shallow container. To condition hair, scoop out enough to massage into the scalp and hair. Wrap your head with plastic wrap for 25 to 30 minutes and shampoo out. Hair will be soft, shiny, and healthy-looking.

Use this conditioning treatment for dry or damaged hair. If you use this conditioning treatment once a month, it will keep your hair in tip-top condition.

Flyaway-Hair Conditioner

¼ cup plain yogurt
1 egg

Whisk the yogurt and egg together well.
Massage the conditioner into the hair
before a shower. Leave it in for 5 minutes.
Rinse well with cool water. Shampoo as
usual. This conditioner gives your hair
body, shine, and control. It also moisturizes
dry hair and gets rid of static.

Deep Conditioner for Dry & Damaged Hair

¼ cup olive oil
1 egg yolk

Mix the olive oil and egg yolk and massage
into the hair. Wrap your hair with plastic
wrap and then wrap a towel around the
plastic to keep it in place. Let the conditioner soak for 20 minutes; then shampoo.

Vinegar Conditioner

peel of 1 lemon
½ cup chamomile flowers
4 cups apple-cider vinegar

Pour apple-cider vinegar over the lemon peel and chamomile flowers into a Mason jar. Seal and let the mixture steep in a sunny window for 2 weeks. Or gently heat the vinegar, pour it over the lemon peel and chamomile flowers, and let the mixture steep for about 1 week. Strain and bottle. To use, apply about 2 tablespoons to your hair's rinse water.

This apple-vinegar rinse helps keep the scalp pH balanced, and may promote hair growth. This rinse works well on oily hair. It leaves hair soft and shiny.

Fennel Conditioner

   2 cups boiling water
   1 tablespoon fennel
   1 tablespoon baking soda

Pour boiling water over the fennel. Cover
and steep for 10 minutes and strain. Add
the baking soda. Pour this over the hair as
a final rinse every day for several weeks,
and then use it once a week. You can also
double or triple the recipe, and store it in
the refrigerator. This recipe will keep for
about 1 week.

   Fennel conditioning rinse is good for oily
hair. It helps balance and get rid of oily
scalp conditions.

Peppermint Dandruff Rinse

1 cup apple-cider vinegar
1 cup chopped fresh or ½ cup dried peppermint
2 cups boiling water

Pour the boiling water over the peppermint, and cover to let the mixture steep overnight. Strain, mix with the vinegar, and bottle. Use ½ cup as a final rinse after shampooing; do not rinse out.

This rinse will help rid you of those embarrassing flakes.

Peppermint Hair Rinse

¼ cup dried peppermint
1 cup boiling water

Pour boiling water over the peppermint. Steep for 20 to 30 minutes or until cool. To use, pour this rinse over the scalp after you've shampooed and massage it in. Do not rinse.

Peppermint stimulates the scalp and has a clean, refreshing scent.

Herbal Hair Rinses
  2 tablespoons lemon juice
  2 tablespoons chamomile, thyme, lavender,
   or rose petals
  4 cups boiling water
  ½ cup witch hazel

Pour the boiling water over the chosen
herb. Cover and steep for 30 minutes.
Strain. Add the witch hazel and lemon
juice. Mix well. Use ½ cup as a final rinse.

Chamomile, thyme, lavender, or rose
petals are good for the skin and hair. Use
this rinse once a week after shampooing to
lighten and soften hair. It will bring out
blonde highlights, especially if you let your
hair dry in the sun. Natural blondes will
find their hair is shinier.

Blonde Highlight Rinse

 4 cups boiling water
 1 cup chamomile flowers
 juice of large lemon

Pour boiling water over the chamomile
flowers. Cover and let steep until cooled.
Mix in lemon juice. Use this as a final
rinse after shampooing. Pour over the hair
several times, catching the rinse in a basin.

 Do this once a month and let hair dry in
the sun. This rinse brings out natural
blonde highlights.

Red Highlight Rinse

  1 cup calendula flowers
  4 cups boiling water

Pour the boiling water over the calendula
flowers and cover. Let the mixture steep
until cool and strain. Use as a final rinse
after shampooing. Catch the rinse in a
basin and repeat several times.

  It's helpful to let the hair dry in the sun.
This rinse brings out natural red highlights
and is well suited to redheads.

Brunette Hair Darkener

8 tablespoons loose or 10 tea bags black tea
4 cups boiling water
1 cup fresh or ½ cup dried rosemary or sage
1 teaspoon lemon juice

Make a strong infusion of black tea, using tea bags or loose tea with boiling water. Pour this hot tea over the rosemary or sage. Strain. Add lemon juice. Use this hair darkener as a final rinse. Catch any rinse in a basin and continue to rinse the hair several times. Over time, your hair will shine with rich color.

This rinse darkens and adds richness to dark hair.

Native American Gray-Hair Secret

¼ cup dried sage
1 cup boiling water
1 black tea bag

Make a strong sage tea, using the dried sage and boiling water. Then continue to steep, adding a black tea bag to the sage tea. Let the tea sit overnight. Use this as a final hair rinse every night until you achieve the desired color. Then use it once a week.

This rinse, popularized by Native Americans, helps return hair to its natural brunette or black color.

Setting Gels & Dressings

Hair dressings and gels have long been with us. Here are a few traditional ones. Of course, a few modern variations, such as use of food coloring from Jell-O and Kool-Aid, are rather recent.

Brilliantine

1 cup vodka
¼ cup castor oil

Mix together well. Pour into a spray bottle. Shake before use. Spray on your hair and comb it in. Let the dressing dry. This will give your hair manageability and shine.

This hair-dressing recipe was popular in the 1940s and early 1950s.

Hair-Styling Lotion

1 cup warm water
2 teaspoons orrisroot powder

Mix the warm water and orrisroot powder until well blended. Pour the styling lotion into a spray bottle. Spritz hair and style.

Check for allergies; some people have reactions to orrisroot. If so, just use plain old aloe-vera gel. It sets hair quickly and leaves a shine. You can also use gelatin. Try the unflavored, colorless gelatin variety. Add this to your final rinse water and it will give your hair body and control.

For novelty, instead of the unflavored gelatin, dissolve a packet of fruit-flavored Jell-O in a little boiling water. Select a color to match your hair. Kool-Aid also works, if you want bizarre color.

Hair Gel

½ cup boiling water
1 tablespoon flaxseeds
6 to 8 drops tea-tree essential oil

Pour boiling water over the flaxseeds. Soak for 15 to 20 minutes and strain. Add the tea-tree essential oil and cool completely. The solution will thicken into a gel. Store it in a closed container and use it as you would any styling gel.

This hair gel is great for keeping a hair style in place.

Stay-in-Place Hair Gel

½ cup Irish moss
3 cups water
¼ cup glycerin

Cover the Irish moss with about 1 cup of water and let it soak for 10 minutes. Strain the Irish moss and dump this water. Next, place the herb in 2 cups of boiling water for 20 minutes. Strain and press the herb while the water is still hot. Use this water and add the glycerin. Mix well. Pour the mixture into several containers.

Irish moss gels really well and makes an excellent hair-styling gel.

FACIAL SCRUBS, MASKS & TONERS

Facial Scrubs

Facial scrubs or cleansers are beneficial since the facial skin is sensitive and prone to blackheads, acne, and other problems. We all would love to have smooth, glowing skin without any hassles—and now you can. Try these homemade cleansers; they promise to give your nutrition-starved skin all it needs and more.

Facial scrubs help rid the skin of the top layer of dead skin cells that we constantly shed. They also help prevent clogged pores.

Cornmeal Face Scrub

¼ cup cornmeal
water

Add enough water to the cornmeal to make a thick paste. Apply this scrub to the face gently; then rinse it off.

Oatmeal Cleansing Bags

½ cup quick-cooking rolled oats
½ cup dried rose petals
1 yard (1 m) muslin
5 feet (150 cm) string
water

You'll need muslin squares. Cut several about the size of a washcloth. Place a small handful of rolled oats and a handful of dried rose petals in the middle of a muslin square. Use scented, old-fashioned roses, grown with no pesticides. Tie the muslin square with rolled oats and roses inside together with string. Place these bags in a large glass jar to keep handy in the bathroom.

To use, simply wet the bag down with warm water, squeeze to get all the "juice," and gently rub it over the face. Rinse and pat dry or use a toner or astringent.

Oatmeal makes a milky-smooth pore cleanser that helps get rid of oily skin. If you squeeze the bags out, you can use them twice. Throw them out after a second use.

Pretty-as-Can-Be Facial Cleanser

2 tablespoons lemon juice
⅓ cup witch hazel
2 tablespoons glycerin
2 tablespoons comfrey-leaf tea

Make a strong tea using 1 tablespoon comfrey leaves and ½ cup boiling water. Let steep for 10 minutes. Mix the lemon juice, witch hazel, glycerin, and 2 tablespoons comfrey tea. Keep the mixture refrigerated. To cleanse, use a cotton ball to apply and rinse off.

This cleanser will help fade spots and freckles.

Many common foods help cleanse and smooth our skin. So, it makes sense to use them outside the body, on the skin, as well as inside it. Here are a few skin cleansers to try. They appear to enrich skin, act as astringents, provide beneficial rather than harmful bacteria, and balance the skin's Ph.

Strawberries: Mash a few strawberries and rub them over the face. The strawberries help clear the complexion and bleach out freckles and age spots.

Tomatoes: Mash a few slices of tomato and rub it over the face. The tomato has astringent action for oily skin.

Eggs: Use the egg yolk. Mix and spread it over the face and rinse it off with warm water. This seems to provide good nutrition for skin.

Cucumber: Rub cucumber slices over the face and rinse. This helps reduce puffiness, especially around the eyes. Let the slices sit over closed eyelids for 5 minutes.

Honey: Honey is great for skin, since it is antiseptic and makes skin soft. Merely spread it over the face in a circular motion. Rinse clean.

Yogurt: Rub plain yogurt into the skin. Make sure it has active yogurt cultures, since they will help balance the skin's pH. Rinse.

Dry Skin Cleansers

These simple cleansers remove makeup and help moisturize skin. They're also helpful for dry, aging skin.

Vegetable Shortening: Believe it or not, vegetable shortening makes a great cleanser. Just place it in a pretty little jar to use in the bathroom.

Vitamin E Oil: Plain vitamin E oil is very healing to skin.

Olive Oil & Vegetable Oil: These help remove makeup and act as moisturizers since they help the skin retain water.
Petroleum Jelly: Just apply petroleum jelly to dry skin and tissue it off.

Milk-Roses Facial Cleanser

4 tablespoons dried rose petals
4 tablespoons powdered milk

In a blender, make the dried rose petals into a powder. Mix with the powdered milk. Place the mixture in a glass jar with a small spoon or scoop. When ready to use, put a small amount of milk-roses cleanser in your palm and mix it with warm water. Apply it as a paste to your face and rub gently in a circular motion. Rinse. Pat the face dry. Milk roses and rosewater are centuries-old favorites for making your skin smooth, glowing, and wrinkle-free.

Almond Gel Cleanser

  2 teaspoons quince seeds
  2 bags peppermint tea
  2 cups distilled water
  ½ cup finely ground raw almonds

Bring the water to boil, adding peppermint
tea bags to make a strong tea. Steep for 5
minutes and remove the tea bags. Now
return the tea to heat, bringing it to a boil,
and add the quince seeds. Reduce the heat
to simmer for 15 minutes. Stir constantly
to prevent scorching. This mixture will gel
quite nicely. Strain out the seeds. Keep the
gel refrigerated.

  To use, keep finely ground almonds in a
plastic bag. Mix some ground almonds
with the gel to form a paste, and gently
apply the paste on the neck and face. Let
it soak into the skin a few minutes; then

rinse with warm water. This gel cleanser is good for all skin types.

Masks

Masks are a great way to refine your complexion and hydrate your skin. They will give you a youthful glow. You can use a facial mask, mixed from ingredients you have on hand, once a week.

Yogurt Oily-Skin Mask

  4 to 6 tablespoons oat flour
  4 drops fresh lemon or lime juice
  small tomato, ½ cucumber, or 4 to 5 strawberries
  ½ cup yogurt with live cultures
  1 teaspoon unscented night cream

To make an oat flour, powder dry rolled oats in a blender. Use just the pulp, with seeds removed, from the tomato or cucumber. If you are using the strawberries instead of the tomato or cucumber, just mash them, seeds and all. A blender or a masher will easily pulverize the cucumber, tomato, or strawberries.

Mix the lemon juice; mashed tomato, cucumber, or strawberries; yogurt; and night cream in a small cup. Add enough oatmeal flour to the mixture to form a thick paste. Apply the facial mask and let dry about 30 minutes. Remove the mask with tissues and rinse with cool water.

Deep-Cleansing Clay Mask

  1 teaspoon water
  1 teaspoon cosmetic clay
  1 drop peppermint essential oil

Combine the water and cosmetic clay to form a paste. Add the peppermint essential oil. Mix well and apply to the face. Let the clay mask dry completely; then rinse it away with warm water.

First test for skin sensitivities. If you are prone to dry skin, use this mask only once a month. Keep the mask well away from the eyes.

❧

Victorian Elegance & Simplicity

Old-Fashioned Egg-White Mask

Victorian ladies used beaten egg white as a favorite facial mask. Just apply beaten egg white to the face and let the mask dry. Then use warm water to rinse it off after 15 to 30 minutes.

Honey & Oatmeal Mask

Honey and rolled oats were used in another popular traditional mask. Grind up the rolled oats in a blender to make a flour. Add a little oat flour to the honey, making the mask the consistency of a thick paste, and spread it over the entire face.

Leave the mask on for 15 to 30 minutes. Tissue off and rinse with cool water.

Cucumber Eyes

While they waited for their egg-white or honey-and-oat masks to dry, Victorian ladies reclined and placed cucumber slices on their eyes. The cucumber slices help reduce puffy eyes and dark circles. The mask brings a rosy glow to cheeks.

Fruit Mask

½ cup boiling water
2 prunes
½ mashed banana
½ cup quick-cooking oats
honey (optional)

Pour the boiling water over the prunes. When the prunes are softened, mash them. Add the rolled oats and mashed banana. Mix well. Cover and let the mixture sit until cool. Add honey if needed for a thick paste. Smear this fruit mask on your face and wait 30 minutes. Then rinse.

This fruit mask softens and moisturizes dry skin. It is also helpful for skin prone to breakouts. You can even eat the leftover mixture as a healthful breakfast!

Cooling Face Mask

 1 egg white
 ¼ cup mayonnaise
 ¼ cup cucumber slices

In a blender, put the egg white, mayonnaise, and cucumber slices. Blend well. Spread the mask on the face and leave for 30 to 60 minutes. Tissue off and rinse the face with cool water.

This cooling face mask is great for dry skin, for bleaching freckles and spots, and for hydrating aging skin.

Egg-Yolk Mask

  1 egg yolk
  1 to 2 teaspoons olive oil
  1 to 2 teaspoons honey

Mix a little warmed honey with the egg
yolk, and add enough olive oil to form a
thick paste. Smear the mask all over the
face and let it dry. Rinse off the mask with
warm water.

  This mask is good for dry skin, and it
helps skin stay smooth and soft. As for the
edible part, you'll probably want to avoid
eating raw eggs.

Skin Toners & Astringents

Toners and astringents help refresh tired skin, clear blemished complexions, and tighten pores.

❦

Peppermint Splash

½ cup witch hazel
¼ cup peppermint tea
6 drops peppermint extract (optional)

Mix the witch hazel, peppermint tea, and peppermint extract. Pour the mixture into a bottle. Shake well.

Shake before using. Pour a little into the hand and splash it onto the face. Avoid getting the toner near or in your eyes. If you don't want to splash, simply apply it with a cotton ball.

Acne-Be-Gone Toner

  1 teaspoon dried or 1 tablespoon fresh sage
    leaves
  1 cup boiling water
  ½ cup apple-cider vinegar

First, make an infusion with sage leaves and the boiling water. Add the apple-cider vinegar. Cool and store in the refrigerator. Apply twice a day with a clean cotton ball.

  Lavender Substitution: This toner helps clear red, inflamed, or pimply skin. For variety, make the same recipe, but substitute lavender buds for the sage.

  Tea Tree Added: Tea-tree essential oil is excellent for clearing up the complexion. Add 10 drops to 1 cup of the sage or lavender-bud tea. Use as directed.

Lemon Astringent

¼ cup lemon juice
½ cup distilled water
⅓ cup witch hazel

Mix the lemon juice, distilled water, and witch hazel well, and pour it into a bottle. Shake the astringent before using it.

To help fade skin spots, use this twice a day. Lemon astringent is very refreshing.

Rose Toner

½ cup rosewater
½ teaspoon tincture of benzoin

To make rosewater, add rose petals to boiling distilled water. Let cool and strain. Add more and more petals until the water has a strong scent that pleases you. Add tincture of benzoin. The mixture will turn milky.

Apply the rose toner twice a day. For dry skin, apply the toner after cleansing. It helps condition skin and helps remove the top layer of dead skin cells, leaving the face smooth.

Oily Skin Toner

1 tablespoon fresh or 2 teaspoons dried rosemary or thyme
1 cup boiling water
½ teaspoon honey
½ teaspoon tincture of benzoin

Make a strong tea with the rosemary or thyme added to boiling water. Let steep 10 minutes. Add honey and tincture of benzoin. Mix well. Bottle and label.

Apply the toner with a clean cotton ball morning and night. This toner tightens pores and returns skin to its normal balance.

Woodland Pine Astringent

  1 cup pine needles
  ½ cup distilled water
  ¼ cup witch hazel

Place water and pine needles in a saucepan
and bring to a boil. Cool and strain. Pour
the solution into a bottle and add the
witch hazel. Store it in the medicine
cabinet.

  Apply the astringent with a cotton ball all
over the face.

FOR THE BATH

What better way to give yourself a bit of luxury than an exotic soak in the tub. Take 20 minutes to float away your cares and woes while you beautify your body. If you make your own bath products, you can afford to luxuriate any time.

Bath Oils & Soaks

Cleopatra's Bath
½ cup powdered milk
½ cup dried, powdered rose petals
handful dried, loose rose petals

Mix the dried milk and rose petals well. Store them in a plastic bag until you're ready to use them. You can mix up a large batch of bath bags to have them on hand.

Add the packet to a warm bath. It will soften skin and make you feel like a queen. Add a few fragrant dried rose petals to float on the water. Pick them out before draining the water.

Relaxing Bath Oil

1 tablespoon red turkey oil
1 drop lavender essential oil
2 drops rose essential oil or 9 drops rose-geranium essential oil

Mix red turkey oil, lavender essential oil, and rose-geranium essential oil. Use 1 tablespoon per bath. Double or triple this recipe to have it on hand.

Red turkey oil, derived from castor oil., mixes completely with water and doesn't just coat the surface of the bathwater. Avoid red turkey oil if allergic.

Refreshing Bath Cream

   2 tablespoons liquid lanolin
   6 drops lemon-verbena essential oil
   4 drops peppermint essential oil

Mix the lanolin, lemon-verbena essential oil, and peppermint essential oil well and add to the bathwater. Soak no longer than 20 minutes. This bath cream is very cooling on a hot day.

Fancy Love Bath

   2 tablespoons olive oil
   6 drops sandalwood essential oil
   3 drops rose essential oil

Mix the olive oil and the sandalwood and rose essential oils into running bathwater. Swirl to mix, and sink in for a nice 20-minute soak.

Ultimate Bath Oil

¾ cup peanut oil
¼ cup olive oil
¼ cup rosewater
40 drops lavender essential oil
20 drops chamomile essential oil
18 drops geranium essential oil

Mix the peanut and olive oil, rosewater, and the lavender, chamomile, and geranium essential oils well. Pour the bath oil mixture into a squeeze bottle. This recipe makes enough for eight baths. Use 2 tablespoons per bath.

This recipe is based on an old remedy used to soften and beautify skin and to get rid of blemishes and marks. I included essential oils for added benefit.

Try these herbs in a strong tea, using about 1 tablespoon fresh or 2 teaspoons dried herb to 1 cup boiling water. Steep for 10 minutes. Then add the herbal tea to your bathwater for a wonderful soak.

❧

Chamomile: soothing to inflamed skin
Lavender: relaxing; relieves mild burns and headaches
Rose Petals: uplifting; balancing; good for aging skin
Mint: invigorating; cooling
Hyssop: calming
Thyme: stimulating; relieves headaches and muscle pain
Eucalyptus: stimulating; aids skin healing; soothes aches and pains; relieves cold symptoms

Bath Foams & Bubbles

Fizzy Bath Salts

½ cup cornstarch
½ cup citric acid
1 cup baking soda
10 drops eucalyptus essential oil
6 drops lemon-verbena essential oil
4 drops peppermint essential oil

Mix the cornstarch, citric acid, baking soda, and the eucalyptus, lemon-verbena, and peppermint essential oils very well. Store the fizzy bath salts in a well-sealed container.

Add 1 cup to the bath. It will bubble and fizz delightfully. This recipe makes two baths.

Sweet Vanilla Bubbles

2 cups olive oil or sweet almond oil
1 cup mild liquid soap
2 tablespoons vanilla extract
½ cup honey

Blend the olive or sweet almond oil, liquid soap, vanilla extract, and honey. Store in a squeeze bottle. Add 2 tablespoons or more per bath.

Lavender Bubble Indulgence

2 cups mild liquid soap
½ cup glycerin
2 teaspoons sugar
40 drops lavender essential oil

Mix the liquid soap, glycerin, sugar, and lavender essential oil well. Use 3 tablespoons per bath for lots of fragrant bubbles.

Sweet Heaven Bubble Bath

1 cup mild, unscented liquid soap
1 cup honey
2 tablespoons olive or sweet-almond oil
2 tablespoons almond extract
2 tablespoons glycerin

Mix the liquid soap, honey, olive or sweet-almond oil, almond extract, and glycerin well. Use 2 tablespoons per bath.

Bath Bags

These bath bags make wonderful scrubbers. Bath bags are easy to use. These simple potions can smooth and beautify skin, relieve sore muscles, banish headaches, or wash away stress. They also make great gifts for anyone who enjoys a relaxing bath or, if you wish, an invigorating soak.

You can make several and store them for bath time. Pack the bath bags into large plastic bags or in a large glass jar and seal.

You can make the bath bags out of muslin, a washcloth, or dish towel, cut into a length that makes 4- to 6-inch squares when folded and sewn. One washcloth can make two small bags. You'll need thread to stitch up the bag and twine or string to tie the bag shut at the top. Leave a loop of twine loose from the bag tie so that you can hang the bag over a spigot. For fancy bags, you may want to add lace and ribbon.

Making the Bag

For the bag, you'll need muslin, cut to washcloth size for each bag, and twine. Place a handful of the desired herbs in the middle of the muslin. Add ½ cup of mild soap flakes. Tie the muslin cloth into a bag, trim the top, and leave enough twine to dangle the bag from the spigot as water fills the tub.

In your bath, swish the bag around, and rub it over the body to cleanse and soap up. When done with your bath, squeeze excess water out of the bag and hang it up to dry. You can use a bath bag about two to three times before disposing of it.

Hint: Buy a small quantity of pretty kitchen towels or bath washcloths in colors that match your décor or that work with particular holidays or seasons.

First, choose a handful of the desired herb(s) for the effect you want.

Oily Skin: eucalyptus leaves, lemongrass, rosemary, thyme

Dry Skin: lavender, chamomile, rose petals

Relaxation: lavender, rose, catnip, hyssop

Invigorating: rosemary, thyme, mint, lemon verbena, basil

Aching Muscles: sage, bay leaves, rosemary

❦

Follow directions for Making the Bag on pp. 218–219.

Rose-Milk Bath Bags

¼ to ½ cup powdered milk
¼ to ½ cup powdered rose petals
3 to 6 drops rose essential oil

For the rose milk, use ¼ to ½ cup powdered milk and add ¼ to ½ cup powdered rose petals. To powder the dried rose petals, use a blender or food processor. Add a few drops of rose essential oil to each bag, if you wish. This luxurious bath bag soothes aging skin and relieves headaches and grief.

Cut muslin into squares that are washcloth size. Make them half as big if you want smaller bags. Fold them in half and sew up the sides to make a little bag. You can make them plain, tying them closed with string, or fancy, adding a drawstring closure and lace.

Lemon-Zing Bath Bag

2 tablespoons grated mild soap
½ cup dried peppermint leaves
16 drops lemongrass essential oil

Cut a washcloth in two to sew two little bags. Mix the grated soap, peppermint leaves, and lemongrass essential oil. Into each bag, put half the recipe. Tie each bag with twine and use it in the tub or shower. These filled bath bags can be used only once. You can keep the washcloth bags and refill them with new ingredients.

Oatmeal Bath Bags

handful rolled oats
handful lavender
10 drops lavender essential oil

In the middle of the cloth, put the rolled oats and lavender buds. You can make the scent stronger by adding 10 drops of lavender essential oil to each baggie.

Tie each bag up with twine and loop the twine so that you can hang it over the faucet or spigot as water fills the tub. Or simply soak the bag with water in the shower and use it as a scrubber. Squeeze and rub the bath bag all over the body.

This milky bath is great for dry skin and soothes itchy skin. Lavender is very relaxing. Each bag can be used twice; just squeeze out excess water and hang it up to dry.

Rose-Petal Bath Bag

handful rose petals
2 to 6 drops rose essential oil (optional)

This bath bag acts more like a tea, since the essential oil from the rose petals is released into the hot bathwater. To make fancy bath bags, tie them in little white muslin bags or rose-colored washcloths. Use pink lace and ribbon, if you like. Add a few drops of rose essential oil to each to make the scent stronger. Leave a few dried rose petals out to float atop the water or use fresh petals from a single rose. Heavenly!

Substitutions: You can substitute mint leaves, chamomile, or rosemary for the rose petals and have a luxurious herbal-tea bath soak any time.

Bath Salts & Powders

Bath salts are a good way to soak out the body's toxins as well as to balance skin pH levels. They leave the skin feeling silky soft and smooth. The herbal body powders help deodorize and make you feel fresh on hot days. They also help heal skin.

Epsom Salts Soak #1

  3 cups Epsom salts
  12 drops or ¼ teaspoon glycerin
  2 to 4 drops food coloring
  10 drops (total) essential oils, your choice

Mix Epsom salts, glycerin, and food coloring until salt crystals are well colored. Put ½ cup of the mixture into separate little plastic bags. To each bag, add up to 10 drops (no more) of soothing essential oil.

You can choose more than one essential

oil, if you wish, but do not exceed the total
of 10 drops for all essential oils combined.
Each bag makes one bath. This bath helps
with achy or tired muscles and sends you
off to a deep sleep.

Epsom Salts Soak #2
   1 cup Epsom salts
   2 cups borax
   1 cup sea salt
   ¼ cup clay powder
   64 drops (total) essential oils, your choice

Mix the Epsom salts, borax, and sea salt
well. Then add the clay powder. Work the
essential oils into the mixture.

Put the ingredients, using ½ cup per bath
bag, in muslin bags with drawstrings or
pretty ribbons. Use one bath bag for your
bath.

Easy Bath Salts

 2 cups Epsom salts
 1 cup baking soda
 1 cup sea salt
 64 drops (total) essential oils, your choice
 3 to 5 drops food coloring (optional)

Mix the Epsom salts, baking soda, sea salt, and essential oils well. Add food coloring, if you wish. Add ½ cup of these easy bath salts to your bathwater and enjoy.

This recipe makes eight baths. Place the bath salts in a pretty, decorative jar and seal tightly. Use a scoop to pour the bath salts into warm bathwater. If the bath salts cake, just use the scoop to break them up.

Substitutions: You can omit the sea salt and use 2 cups baking soda instead of 1 cup baking soda and 1 cup sea salt.

After-Bath Dusting Powders

Healing Body & Foot Powder

 1 cup powdered cosmetic clay
 1 cup powdered arrowroot
 2 tablespoons powdered lavender buds
 2 tablespoons powdered peppermint leaves
 40 drops tea-tree essential oil

Blend the lavender buds and the peppermint leaves in a blender. Mix the cosmetic clay and arrowroot with the lavender buds and peppermint leaves. Add the tea-tree essential oil and mix completely.

Store this healing body and foot powder in a sealed jar. Apply it to clean skin as needed or twice a day. It helps reduce body odor and relieves rashes and athlete's foot.

Herbal Dusting Powder

  2 cups cosmetic clay powder
  2 cups slippery-elm powder
  2 cups cornstarch
  2 cups powdered rose petals
  40 drops (total) essential oils

In a large bowl, mix the cosmetic clay, slippery elm, cornstarch, and rose petals. Work in the essential oils of your choice, using no more than 40 drops total.

Store this herbal powder in sealed jars with a large cotton ball or powder puff. Dust the body liberally after the baths to scent. The powder also absorbs perspiration.

SLEEP POTIONS
& DREAM PILLOWS

Sleepy Teas

Herbal teas have enjoyed a long history. Originally, these teas were brewed for medicinal purposes, not for pleasure. Their pleasing tastes were simply an added bonus. Fortunately, they are very healing, and many herbs can help you relax or indeed help send you off to dreamland. Since many of us have trouble getting to sleep from time to time, it's nice to be able to reach for a warm cup of herbal tea to aid us. Choose an herb or blend that suits your taste. Consult the list of Popular Sleepy-Tea Herbs on p. 232.

Some teas rise and fall in popularity. Catnip was a favorite tea in England before Chinese teas, like the familiar black *Camellia* varieties, were introduced.

How to Prepare Herbal Teas

When making an herbal tea, begin with fresh water. Bring the water to a boil, toss in 2 teaspoons fresh or 1 teaspoon dry herb for each cup brewed. Remove from heat and let steep covered for 5 to 10 minutes. Strain and sweeten with honey, if you wish.

❧

Simples

A simple herbal blend consists of one type of herb brewed and sipped. Perhaps you favor chamomile with its fruity, applelike taste or lavender with its sweet, exotic taste (my favorite).

Drink no more than 3 cups per day. The best time of day to drink sleepy-time tisanes is at the end of the day, right before bed-time.

❦

Popular Sleepy-Tea Herbs

Try one of these herbs in boiling water to make a tea when you want to get to sleep.

Chamomile: calms and relaxes.
Catnip: acts as a sedative.
Lavender: relieves migraines; relaxes; sedates.
Lemon Balm: refreshes body and mind; helps reduce anxiety, depression, and nervousness.
Rose: calms the mind and body; reduces stress; encourages sleep.
Sage: calms nerves; banishes headaches.
Sweet Marjoram: calms; warms; helps relieve insomnia, tension, and headaches.
Valerian Root: acts as a tranquilizer; helps relieve insomnia, frayed nerves, and migraine headaches.

Softly-to-Sleep Tea Blend

½ cup dried chamomile flowers
½ cup dried lemon balm
¼ cup dried catnip

Blend the chamomile, lemon balm, and catnip well. To help you sleep, use 1 teaspoon per cup of boiling water. Sip slowly. Store the tea in a tightly sealed jar.

Sleepless Nights Tea Blend

½ cup dried chamomile
½ cup dried sweet marjoram
¼ cup dried thyme
¼ cup dried sage

Blend the dried herbs chamomile, sweet marjoram, thyme, and sage. Store the tea in a sealed container. Use 1 teaspoon per cup boiling water. Sweeten to taste.

❦

Magic Nights Tea Blend
1 cup dried lavender
1 cup dried peppermint
1 cup dried rose petals
1 teaspoon nutmeg

Blend the lavender, peppermint, rose petals, and nutmeg well. Store the tea in a sealed bag or jar. This tea is very tasty and soothing. Before bed, brew a cup of tea with 1 teaspoon of this herbal mix with 1 cup boiling water.

Valerian Sedative Tea

½ teaspoon powdered valerian root
cinnamon stick or ⅛ teaspoon cinnamon
1 cup boiling water
honey (optional)

Pour the boiling water over the valerian
root. Cover and let steep for 10 minutes.
Strain and add the cinnamon and honey to
taste. This tea is for when you really need
to get to sleep. Be careful not to overuse it.
Overdosing can cause the opposite reaction. It's best to sip just 1 or 2 cups on rare
occasions.

Dream Pillows

Especially popular in the Victorian era, dream pillows were made with silks and fancy laces. The herbs inside lent their scents and helped lull people off to dreamland. You can make your dream pillows as elaborate or as plain as you wish. Gentle herbs with pleasing scents, like lavender, chamomile, and rose, are good for making dream pillows for children. They seem to help banish nightmares.

Dream Pillow Basics

You'll need some fabric and dried herbs. You want to create a small, flat pillow that can be slipped between the pillowcase of the sleeper's regular pillow. Decorate it as you wish. Add enough herbs to make a flat pouch, and, if you wish, add 5 to 10 drops of a corresponding essential oil before sewing the pillow closed.

Lavender Dream-Pillow Mix

  6 tablespoons lavender buds
  6 drops sandalwood essential oil
  4 drops ylang-ylang essential oil

For this pillow, add sandalwood and ylang-ylang essential oils to the lavender buds. This pillow mix will encourage a deep, relaxing sleep and good dreams.

Psychic Dream-Pillow Blend #1

  1 part rosemary
  1 part valerian
  1 part hops
  1 part jasmine

Mix equal amounts of the dried herbs and fill your dream pillow. This pillow helps you sleep deeply and soundly, banishes headaches, and encourages psychic dreams.

Psychic Dream-Pillow Blend #2

½ cup sweet marjoram
¼ cup mugwort
1 teaspoon cloves
5 drops frankincense essential oil

Mix the sweet marjoram, mugwort, and cloves. Add the frankincense essential oil. This blend encourages prophetic dreams and visions.

Nervous Nellie Dream Pillow

¾ cup lavender
¼ cup bergamot
¼ cup rose petals
4 to 5 drops ylang-ylang essential oil

Mix the dried lavender, bergamot, rose petals, and ylang-ylang essential oil. Stuff a little pillow. This dream pillow helps soothe frazzled nerves.

Dream-Pillow Blend

  ½ cup sweet woodruff
  ¼ cup lavender
  2 tablespoons hops
  2 tablespoons rosebuds
  2 tablespoons rosemary
  1 teaspoon cinnamon or orrisroot powder

Blend the sweet woodruff, lavender, hops, rosebuds, and rosemary. Add the cinnamon or orrisroot powder. Slip the herbal blend into little pillows.

Relax for a soothing sleep.

Knockout Dream Pillow

¾ cup dried chamomile flowers
¼ cup dried clary sage
4 drops clary-sage essential oil
3 drops jasmine essential oil

Mix the dried chamomile flowers and dried clary sage. Add the clary-sage and jasmine essential oils. Use this pillow for those nights when nothing else will do.

Eye Pillows

These little pillows are made to lie across the eyes (4×10 inches or 10×25 cm). Eye pillows are great when you have eyestrain or want to take a short nap. They also block out light, and the relaxing scent of the herbs helps, too.

Lavender Eye Pillows

¼ cup lavender buds
¼ cup flaxseed or rose petals
4 to 6 drops essential oil

For a great eye pillow, mix equal amounts of lavender buds with flaxseed. Add a few drops of essential oil of your choice.

Substitutions: You can substitute rose petals for the flaxseed. You could also mix half lavender with half rose petals and keep the flaxseed. Add a few drops of essential oil(s), if you wish.

Sleep Salves

These sleep salves or rubs help you get to sleep. They work when the skin absorbs the properties of the herbs and essential oils.

❧

Dreamy Cream
  ½ cup olive oil
  2 teaspoons melted beeswax
  1 teaspoon mugwort
  ½ teaspoon rosemary
  ½ teaspoon spearmint
  ½ teaspoon sage
  ½ teaspoon lavender
  2 capsules or ¼ teaspoon vitamin E oil

Gently warm the olive oil. Add the dried mugwort, rosemary, spearmint, sage, and lavender. Let steep overnight. Strain. Heat gently, adding the beeswax to the mixture

and melting it. Remove from heat. Add
the vitamin E oil and pour the salve into
containers to harden. At bedtime, rub the
salve into your temples to encourage sleep.

❧

Lavender Oil Rub
   2 cups peanut oil
   1 cup lavender buds

Place lavender buds in the peanut oil and
seal the jar. Set in a sunny window for 1
week, shaking regularly. Strain. Rub the
lavender oil into the temples, neck, and
hands before bedtime to help send you to
sleep.

Warming Orange & Lavender Rub

  2 tablespoons warmed vegetable oil
  5 drops lavender essential oil
  5 drops sweet-orange essential oil

Warm the vegetable oil. Add the lavender and sweet-orange essential oils. Rub the oil into the temples before slipping into bed.

Calming Carbohydrates

Scientists have recently discovered that carbohydrates (refined carbohydrates seem to work best) help calm body and mind and can put us to sleep. You need just an ounce or two (30 to 60 g) of carbohydrates to do the trick, though it takes about 20 minutes for the effects to set in.

Protein, eaten in late evening, may keep us awake. Protein is helpful when you need to be alert, say, for an important meeting.

⁂

Onion Sandwich Sleep Remedy

thinly sliced onion
2 slices bread
butter

A traditional remedy for insomnia is to eat a thinly sliced onion between two slices of buttered bread shortly before bedtime.

More Sleep Remedies

Wet-Towel Sleep Cure

In the summer heat, wet a towel with cool water and wrap it around the head. Lie down. This is helpful when you are over-heated, since it both cools you down and relaxes you.

Hops Sleep Bitters

½ cup hops
4 tablespoons orange peel
2 teaspoons cardamom
2 teaspoons cinnamon
½ teaspoon cloves
1 cup vodka
4 cups sherry wine
1 cup simple syrup
water

Soak the hops, orange peel, cardamom, cinnamon, and cloves in the vodka and sherry for 1 week. Strain and add the syrup and enough water to make 1 gallon (or about 3.8 liters). Mix well and seal. Use as needed.

Sip a wineglass of the bitters at bedtime.

Quieting Children

Mellow Scents

2 to 6 drops clary-sage or lavender
essential oil

Place a few drops of clary-sage essential oil
on a cotton ball, and place it underneath
the pillowcase. You can also put a few
drops of lavender essential oil on the collar
of a child's pajamas to slow the child down
and send him to sleep.

Milk & Honey Soother

small glass buttermilk
1 teaspoon honey

To calm a hyperactive child over age three,
warm some buttermilk and mix in 1 teaspoon of honey. Have the child drink this
before bedtime.

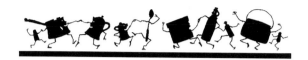

Part 3
PET CARE

In this part, you'll find remedies designed to ease your pet's simple ills. You'll also learn ways to prevent and protect your pet against fleas and other parasites. You'll delight in recipes for homemade goodies for the dogs, cats, or birds in your life. Other easy-to-make products will enhance your pet's appearance. Catnip toys will intrigue your cat. You'll discover remedies to help your canary, parakeet, or parrot feel tops. Wild bird feed will bring more birds to your windows.

Remember that for pets, a little goes a long way. Give them very small amounts of the remedies, as directed. Also do not give a small cat, dog, or bird the same amount you would a larger one. Kittens and puppies would take a half dose of any grown-up pet remedy.

Animals do not respond the same way humans do to certain substances. For instance, animals react badly to tea-tree essential oil, although it has been found in many books as a topical remedy for both humans and animals.

Do not give a cat aspirin, willow, or yarrow, since all contain salicylates, which can be fatal for cats. Cats must also be kept away from some plants, like oleander.

REMEDIES FOR CATS

Arthritis & Rheumatism

Older cats may suffer from arthritis or rheumatism. You can give them a little relief with these remedies.

Comfrey Juice

    2 cups boiling water
    3 to 4 comfrey leaves
    1 teaspoon dried or 1 tablespoon fresh hops
    leaves

Pour the boiling water over the comfrey leaves. Add the dried or fresh hops leaves. Let the mixture soak. Strain. Give your cat 20 to 30 drops in water for pain.

Valerian Pain Tincture

1 teaspoon valerian root
1 tablespoon St.-John's-wort leaves
1 cup distilled water
½ cup honey

Bring the water to boil and add valerian root. Let simmer for 10 minutes. Remove the pot from heat. Add St.-John's-wort. Let cool. Mix well with the honey. To use, add 20 drops to the cat's water or to a little milk as needed.

Catnip Tea

1 teaspoon dried or 2 teaspoons fresh catnip
1 cup boiling water

Make a catnip tea as you normally would, using fresh or dried catnip and boiling water. Steep for 5 minutes. Pour out 2 tablespoons to cool for kitty to relieve pain.

You can drink the rest, and both of you will feel much better. Soothing catnip tea aids digestion and relieves pain. It relaxes and calms humans, too. Catnip, as you've probably discovered, acts like a narcotic for cats. Your feline will love this.

❧

Old Cats' Balm-of-Gilead Rub

½ cup balm of Gilead buds
water
4 (400 I.U.) capsules or ½ teaspoon vitamin
  E oil

Pour boiling water over the balm of Gilead buds, using just enough to cover the herb well. Let cool and strain. It will become a gel-like substance. Add the vitamin E oil and mix well. To use, rub the gel into affected areas and along the spine. Store in a closed container.

Sometimes as we age, our joints become stiff and painful. The same thing can be true for cats. You can massage this rub into the cat's spine and hind legs to relieve the stiffness. It's OK if the cat licks this mixture, since that will enhance its effects.

Allergies

Cat Anti-Itch Lotion
  1 teaspoon dried comfrey
  1 teaspoon dried goldenseal
  1 teaspoon dried myrrh
  1 teaspoon dried elder
  ½ teaspoon cayenne pepper
  1 cup boiling water
  1 cup aloe-vera juice

Mix the dried comfrey, goldenseal, myrrh, and elder. Add the cayenne pepper. Pour the boiling water over the herb mixture, cover, and let cool. Add the aloe-vera juice. Mix well. Rub into affected areas.

This remedy is good for itching and fur loss caused by fleas and contact allergies.

Castor Oil Allergy Cure

With the evening meal, add 4 drops of cold-pressed, cold-processed castor oil on top of the cat's food until you see a change. This helps cleanse the system of toxins and helps cure any type of allergy. It will also make the cat's coat nice and shiny.

Do not continue more than 2 weeks.

Garlic & Goldenseal Cure

  2 tablespoons powdered garlic
  2 tablespoons powdered goldenseal
  ¼ cup olive oil

Mix the powdered garlic and goldenseal well. Add the olive oil and blend. Add 20 to 30 drops to the cat's food every evening until you see results. This tonic will help balance and support your cat's immune system so that allergies won't be a problem.

Kidney Disorders

You'll know your cat is having problems if you notice a change in the cat's frequency or desire to eliminate. A clue is if the cat begins urinating in strange places, outside the litter box. If you suspect this is the problem, give the cat this tonic in its water for a week. To keep things going smoothly, dose the cat once a month or so.

Cornsilk Kidney Strengthener

2 tablespoons burdock root
2 cups water
2 tablespoons garlic powder
handful fresh or dried corn silk

Add the burdock root to the water and boil for 10 minutes. Remove from heat and add the garlic powder and corn silk. Cover and let cool for 20 minutes. Strain. Add 2 tablespoons to the cat's drinking water each day until symptoms are gone.

This remedy banishes all feline urinary-tract problems.

Digestion & Fur Balls

When your cat is not feeling well and becomes lethargic, you can give it a digestive aid. Cats, because of their grooming habits, have trouble with fur balls. Fur balls give cats constipation and a generally yucky feeling. Try the fur ball treatment here.

Fur Ball Treatment

½ teaspoon olive oil or petroleum jelly

Add ½ teaspoon of olive oil nightly to the food. Or, take a dab of Vaseline petroleum jelly and place on the front paw. Many cats love petroleum jelly and lick it off the paw; this will help ease the fur ball out of the cat's system. You can also use this treatment for prevention.

Fennel & Chamomile Digestive Aid

1 teaspoon fennel seeds
1 teaspoon dried or 2 teaspoons fresh
  chamomile
1 cup boiling water

Pour the boiling water over the fennel
seeds and chamomile. Cover and steep for
10 minutes. Strain and mix well.

Use this digestive aid when you notice
that your cat is not eating well or becoming lethargic. Mix 1 tablespoon with a little olive oil and tuna and feed it to your
pet. It will help relieve constipation and
other digestive ills.

Wounds, Skin Ailments & Ear Mites

Calendula & Lavender Skin Ointment

  1 teaspoon calendula petals
  1 teaspoon lavender buds
  2 tablespoons peanut oil
  2 tablespoons vitamin E oil

Cover the calendula petals and lavender
buds with the peanut oil and vitamin E oil.
Place the mixture in a sunny window and
steep for 2 weeks. Strain. Rub on the cat's
wounds and problem skin.

Sulfur Ointment

  powdered sulfur
  vegetable shortening

Mix equal amounts of powdered sulfur and
vegetable shortening. Store this in a closed
container and keep it handy for emergen-

cies. Rub a little ointment into the cat's wounds, sores, or problem skin to promote quick healing.

This ointment is also good for dogs, cows, horses, or almost any animal.

Ear Mite Remedy
handful wormwood
½ cup warmed olive oil

Place the wormwood in the warmed olive oil. Let steep several days. Strain. Dip a cotton swab into this oil and swab the ear lightly to get rid of ear mites.

You can tell if there's a problem with ear mites if your cat's ear is dirty-looking and red or inflamed.

Sore Paw Relief

 aloe-vera leaf
 castor oil

For sore paws, split an aloe-vera leaf and rub over the pads. You can also rub castor oil into the pads to help heal the skin.

Respiratory Disorders

If your cat has caught a cold and you find him or her sneezing, take action right away.

Thyme Tea

 1 tablespoon thyme
 ½ cup boiling water
 honey

Make a tea of thyme, using the thyme and boiling water. Mix with a little honey and give the cat 1 teaspoon twice a day for congestion.

Cold Congestion Rub

eucalyptus essential oil

Use 1 drop eucalyptus essential oil for each footpad. Rub the eucalyptus essential oil into the cat's footpads twice a day.

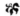

Chest Congestion Remedy

4 drops thyme essential oil
1 teaspoon powdered ginger
1 tablespoon linseed meal

Mix the thyme essential oil, ginger, and linseed meal with a little water to form a bunch of little pills. Set the pills aside to dry and store them in a sealed plastic bag. Give your cat one pill each night until you see improvement.

Cat's Room Mist

  3 drops frankincense essential oil
  2 drops eucalyptus essential oil
  2 drops hyssop essential oil

Cats are very sensitive to scent; go easy.
You can use a diffuser, room humidifier,
steam vaporizer, or electric potpourri burner to scent the air.

  Enclose the cat in a room, and set up
your method for getting the scent into the
air. Add the frankincense, eucalyptus, and
hyssop essential oils to the water of an
electric potpourri burner. Let the burner
run for an hour.

  Try this once a day for several days. The
cat should find the scent relaxing, and it
should help ease your pet's breathing.

Eye Infections

Eyebright

¼ cup dried eyebright
1 cup vodka

Make a tincture by adding the dried eyebright to vodka. Let the mixture sit in a sunny window for 2 weeks. Strain with a coffee filter.

To treat your cat's eye problems, dilute this tincture in a little water, and apply to the eye with an eyedropper. Apply twice a day until symptoms disappear.

This is helpful for pink eye and other eye infections.

Cat's Eye Wash

2 tablespoons comfrey root
2 tablespoons bruised fennel seeds
1 cup distilled water

Bring the water to a boil and add the comfrey root and fennel seeds. Remove from heat. Cover and let steep until cool. Strain. To use, apply several drops in each eye daily until you notice improvement.

After you prepare the eye wash, keep it refrigerated. Let the eye wash come to room temperature before applying it to your cat's eyes.

Fungus & Mange

Tobacco & Salt Treatment

  4 cups boiling water
  4 tablespoons tobacco
  ⅜ cup table salt

You can also try this remedy. Bring the water to boil. Add the tobacco, reduce heat, and simmer. Strain. Add the table salt and mix well. Bottle and label. Wash the area of hair loss and rub this lotion into the skin well.

  This treatment helps rid your pet of fungal infections and mange.

REMEDIES FOR DOGS

Arthritis & Rheumatism

Old dogs, just like you and me, can with injury or age develop stiff, inflamed joints and move painfully.

Dog's Pain Reliever

   2 cups water
   1 tablespoon valerian root
   2 tablespoons fenugreek seeds
   2 tablespoons chamomile
   ½ cup aloe-vera juice

Bring the water and valerian root to a boil and boil for 10 minutes. Remove from heat. Add fenugreek seeds and chamomile. Steep until cool. Strain. Add the aloe-vera juice. Pour ¼ cup of this pain reliever into the dog's drinking water.

This pain reliever is good for older dogs that have trouble getting around because of stiff joints. It helps relieve pain and inflammation.

❧

Dog's White-Willow Arthritis Rub

1 tablespoon white-willow leaves
½ cup witch hazel
4 drops rosemary essential oil
2 drops lavender essential oil

Place the willow leaves in the witch hazel and let steep for 2 weeks. Strain. Add the rosemary and lavender essential oils and mix well.

To use, rub on the dog's spine, hips, and legs. Be gentle and careful as you massage the muscles well. It's good to have this arthritis rub on hand. Do not use for cats.

Dog's Vinegar & Herb Arthritis Rub

  1 tablespoon St.-John's-wort
  1 tablespoon rosemary
  2 tablespoons cayenne pepper
  4 cups apple-cider vinegar

Bring the apple-cider vinegar to a gentle boil. Add the St.-John's-wort, rosemary, and cayenne pepper and remove from heat. Cover, let cool, and strain.

  Rub into affected areas twice daily or when you notice that the animal is stiff or in pain.

Dog's Pain-Relieving Cream

½ cup or more boiling water
2 tablespoons licorice root
2 tablespoons yarrow
2 tablespoons balm of Gilead buds
2 to 3 capsules (¼ to ⅜ teaspoon) vitamin E oil
2 to 6 tablespoons vegetable shortening

Pour enough boiling water over the licorice root, yarrow, and balm of Gilead buds to submerge them. Cover and let cool. Strain and squeeze out the liquid. Add vitamin E oil. Whip this mixture with enough vegetable shortening to make a thick cream.

Massage into the dog's spine and hips to help relieve pain. Rub in well or else this cream can be messy.

Allergies & Itching

For allergies and itching from a host of causes, try one of these remedies.

Dog's Itchy Skin Relief

   6 cups water
   4 tablespoons St.-John's-wort
   4 tablespoons tobacco
   2 cups limewater

Bring the water, St.-John's-wort, and tobacco to a boil. Reduce heat to simmer for 15 minutes. Strain. Add the limewater. Mix well and apply to freshly washed hot spots or inflamed areas.

This helps heal itchy skin, hot spots, or sores caused by mange.

Itching Relief

olive or peanut oil
thyme or rosemary

Fill a Mason jar half-full of olive or peanut oil. To this, add as much thyme or rosemary as the oil will cover. Let steep for 2 weeks. Strain. Rub into the dog's itchy skin. This remedy helps heal inflamed, itching skin, and it prevents infections from scratches.

Bee Pollen Remedy

bee pollen

If you suspect allergies, you can try feeding your dog ½ teaspoon of bee pollen in the dog's food every day. Bee pollen is full of vitamins and minerals.

Anti-Allergy Tonic

   2 cups vinegar
   4 tablespoons cod liver oil
   2 tablespoons powdered garlic
   5 tablespoons desiccated liver powder
   4 tablespoons bonemeal powder

Mix the vinegar, cod liver oil, garlic, liver powder, and bonemeal well. Refrigerate. Shake before use. Mix 3 tablespoons into the dog's daily food rations.

Digestion

Any animal can benefit from dill. It helps release excess gas while easing upset stomachs. Peppermint is also helpful for upset stomachs.

Dill Digestive Tea

1 teaspoon dried or 1 tablespoon fresh dill weed

1 cup boiling water

Pour boiling water over the dill weed. Let this cool to room temperature and strain. Add ¼ to ½ cup of the dill tea, depending upon the animal's size, to the drinking water.

Substitution: You can substitute peppermint for the dill, since it is a good digestive and helps calm nervous stomachs.

Aloe-Vera Digestion Tonic

2 tablespoons comfrey leaves
2 tablespoons red clover
2 tablespoons chamomile
½ cup distilled water, enough to cover herbs
½ cup or more aloe-vera juice

Bring water to boil and pour over the comfrey leaves, red clover, and chamomile. Cover and let cool. Strain. Add the aloe-vera juice in an amount equal to that of the herbal liquid and mix well. Refrigerate. Squirt 2 droppers of this down the dog's throat twice a day.

This tonic helps reduce all digestive problems as well as constipation.

Peach-Bark Vomiting Remedy

4 cups water
1 cup shredded peach-tree bark

Bring the water to a boil and add the peach-tree bark. Reduce heat to simmer for 15 minutes. Steep covered until cool. Strain and refrigerate.

Add ½ cup of this peach-bark tea to 1 cup water. Encourage the animal to drink if it is weak. Repeat up to three times daily.

If the digestion is very upset or your dog has been ill and you need to control vomiting, this is a helpful remedy.

Wounds, Skin Ailments & Ear Infections

Old Wound Remedy
  grated carrots or mashed turnips
  powdered charcoal

Apply grated carrots to the wound or
scratch twice a day. Boiled, mashed
turnips, applied twice a day, are also good
for healing a dog's wounds. You can also
add powdered charcoal to the grated carrots or mashed turnips.

❧

Calendula Wash
  2 cups distilled water
  1 tablespoon calendula petals
  1 tablespoon echinacea
  1 tablespoon St.-John's-wort

Bring water to boil, add the calendula

petals, echinacea, and St-John's-wort. Remove from heat. Cover, let cool, and strain. Use a cotton ball to daub over the dog's sores, wounds, and scrapes.

This wash helps heal open wounds and nerve endings and prevents infections.

❦

Sore Footpad Remedy (Dogs Only)

handful white-willow bark, twigs, or leaves
water

Place a handful of white-willow bark, twigs, or leaves in a pan. Cover the white willow with water and bring to a boil. Remove from heat and allow the mixture to steep until cool. Strain. To use, apply with a cotton ball to your dog's sore footpads or to clean wounds and sores. Do not use this on cats.

Caution: Willow has the same pain-relieving properties as aspirin. However, willow, like aspirin, can be fatal to cats. This is also true of yarrow and other herbs containing salicylic acid. So, only use willow or yarrow for your dog.

✿

Yarrow & Thyme Healing Drops

2 tablespoons glycerin
3 drops yarrow essential oil
3 drops thyme essential oil

Mix the glycerin and essential oils well. Using a dropper, apply to wounds.

This remedy helps the dog's wounds heal very fast, and it gets rid of infection. Do not use this remedy for cats.

Wart Remedies

tar, basil leaf, or tea-tree essential oil

Sometimes dogs and other animals get warts, just as humans do. Warts are said to be caused by a virus. Here are some old-time cures.

Farmers have traditionally used tar. Daub some tar on the wart; often a second application is not needed.

Instead of using tar, you can rub the wart with a basil leaf twice a day. Or give the animal a few drops of tea-tree essential oil in its drinking water every day.

Mullein Ear Drops

   2 tablespoons mullein
   2 to 4 tablespoons olive oil
   1 capsule or ⅛ teaspoon vitamin E oil

Place the mullein in a small jar and cover it with olive oil. Let the mixture steep in a sunny window for 2 weeks. Strain and add vitamin E. Put several drops in the dog's infected ear.

These ear drops heal any type of ear infection. Ear infections are easy to spot. There may be an odor, discharge, or secretion. The animal may shake its head or rub the infected ear.

Castor Oil Drops: As an alternate remedy, you can add 3 to 6 drops of cold-pressed, cold-processed castor oil into the ear. It heals infections in no time.

Kidney Infections

If you don't walk your dog often enough, it may develop kidney or bladder infections.

Plantain Kidney Tonic

  handful plantain leaves
  2 cups boiling water

Place a small handful of plantain leaves in boiling water. Cover and steep for 30 minutes. Strain and add ¼ cup of this plantain tea to drinking water. Do this daily until symptoms disappear.

 This tonic is great for kidney or bladder infections. It acts as a tonic and has high amounts of the needed, healing minerals.

Respiratory Disorders

Eucalyptus Chest Rub for Dogs

   2 tablespoons peanut oil
   5 drops eucalyptus essential oil
   2 drops peppermint essential oil
   2 drops lavender essential oil

Mix the peanut oil and the eucalyptus, peppermint, and lavender essential oils. Place a small amount of the chest rub on the palm of your hand and rub it into the dog's chest as well as behind the ears.

Eucalyptus Inhaler

   eucalyptus leaves

Make a small pillow of eucalyptus leaves to lay in the dog's bed. Your dog will inhale the cleansing, antiseptic aroma as it sleeps. Eucalyptus opens breathing passages.

Cold & Cough Remedy for Dogs

2 cups apple-cider vinegar
2 tablespoons goldenseal
2 tablespoons licorice root
2 tablespoons thyme
2 crushed garlic cloves
2 cups honey

Soak the herbs in apple-cider vinegar for at least 2 weeks. Strain. Add the honey. When you notice your dog cough or have congestion, place about 2 tablespoons of this over a small amount of food. Dose the animal several times a day. Use less for small dogs.

Fungus & Ringworm

Chamomile & Lavender Antifungal Wash

   1 cup boiling water
   2 chamomile tea bags
   2 drops lavender essential oil
   1 cup honey

Make chamomile tea using 2 tea bags and the boiling water. Let the tea cool to room temperature. Add the honey and the lavender essential oil. Apply this remedy to ringworm or other fungal infections, freely.

Try to apply this to your dog's infection three times a day until it's gone. Honey adds healing power to the essential oil.

Herbal Antifungal Ointment

1 tablespoon comfrey
1 tablespoon goldenseal
1 tablespoon elder
1 tablespoon thyme
½ cup boiling water
3 drops myrrh essential oil
½ cup aloe-vera juice
2 to 6 tablespoons vegetable shortening

Pour enough boiling water over the comfrey, goldenseal, elder, and thyme just to cover them. Cover the pot, let cool, and strain. Add the myrrh essential oil. Measure and add an equal amount of aloe-vera juice. Whip in a little vegetable shortening; use enough to form a cream.

Dab this onto fungal infections.

FLEAS & PARASITES ON CATS & DOGS

Fleas & Insects

Dog Flea Powder

- ½ cup rue
- ½ cup wormwood
- ½ cup lemongrass
- ½ cup chrysanthemum
- ½ cup pennyroyal
- 1 cup baking soda
- 3 or 4 drops pennyroyal essential oil

Powder the rue, wormwood, lemongrass, chrysanthemum, and pennyroyal in a blender. Add the baking soda and pennyroyal essential oil. Make sure everything is well mixed. Store the dog flea powder in a closed container and use as needed. Dust liberally on your dog to discourage fleas.

Cat Flea Powder

½ cup rosemary
½ cup lemongrass
½ cup chrysanthemum
1 cup baking soda
2 to 4 drops pennyroyal essential oil

Powder the rosemary, lemongrass, and chrysanthemum in a blender. Add the baking soda and the pennyroyal essential oil. Store in a closed container.

Apply this powder liberally to the cat to banish fleas.

Lavender Insect Repellant

½ cup distilled water
24 drops lavender essential oil

Mix the water and essential oil well and pour the mixture into a spray bottle. Spray the cat or dog to repel pests. Be careful not to get the spray into the animal's eyes. This spray repels flies, gnats, and fleas.

Spicy Insect Repellant

2 teaspoons peppermint
2 teaspoons thyme
2 cups boiling water
2 cinnamon sticks

With 1 cup boiling water for each 2 teaspoons of herb, make concentrated, double-strength peppermint and thyme teas. Mix the teas and place two cinnamon sticks in the peppermint-thyme tea. Cover and let cool overnight. In the morning, remove the cinnamon sticks and pour the liquid into a spray bottle.

Use this spray to spritz the cat or dog bothered by flies, fleas, or other insects. It will repel pests.

Pine Oil Rub for Dog's Fleas

handful pine needles
½ cup olive oil

Add enough pine needles to be covered by
the olive oil. Let the pine needles soak for
2 weeks in a sunny window. Strain and use
as a skin rub to deter fleas.

Use a small amount of oil in your palm
and rub it into the dog's spine and other
affected areas.

❦

Cedar or Lavender Flea Rub

3 to 6 drops cedarwood essential oil or
lavender essential oil

Place a few drops of cedarwood or lavender essential oil on a soft cloth and rub
over the cat's or dog's fur.

Cedar & Lavender Flea Shampoo

  4 drops cedarwood essential oil
  4 drops lavender essential oil
  shampoo
  warm water

Add the cedarwood and lavender essential oils to a small pail of warm water with a little shampoo. Swish to disperse the essential oils.

  Dip the animal's brush into this water, and run the brush through the fur to groom and remove fleas. Dip the brush frequently to rinse the brush of fleas; the fleas should die in the water.

Orange Flea Rinse

fresh or dried orange peel
water

Use fresh or dried orange peels. Place the rinds of chopped orange peel in a large pan and cover them with water. Bring to a boil. Cook until the orange rinds are soft. Remove from heat, cover, and cool to room temperature. Strain and use as a final refreshing rinse when bathing the dog or cat. Use once a week during flea season.

Rosemary Flea Dip for Dogs

1 cup fresh rosemary
4 cups boiling water

Pour boiling water over the rosemary and let the mixture steep until cool. Strain and pour this flea dip over the dog as a final rinse. Leave the rosemary rinse on your pet.

Garlic: Add the contents of 1 or 2 garlic capsules to the pet's food during flea season. Most pets love garlic; fleas hate garlic. Or you can grind fresh garlic to mix with the food.

Vitamin B$_1$: Grind a 100-mg tablet of vitamin B$_1$ (thiamine) into a powder (or simply open a capsule) and add it to your pet's food daily.

Apple-Cider Vinegar: Apple-cider vinegar added to the pet's water helps repel insects and makes the animal healthy.

Homemade Flea Collars

  1 teaspoon alcohol
  2 drops lavender essential oil
  2 drops pennyroyal essential oil
  2 drops thyme essential oil
  2 drops cedarwood essential oil

Mix the alcohol and the lavender, penny-royal, thyme, and cedarwood essential oils in a small dish; then soak the pet's collar in the solution. Remove and spread the collar out to dry in the bathtub or sink over-night. Then place it around your pet's neck.

You can also soak the collar in alcohol and garlic oil, but the garlic scent will be strong. You can buy a plain, cloth collar fairly cheaply and treat it yourself once a month.

It's good to dip dogs in an antiflea solution; then tie on an herbal flea collar. Since cats dislike bathing, collars would be best for them.

Treating Pet Bedding for Fleas

Pennyroyal Flea Treatment
fresh or dried pennyroyal
lavender essential oil

If your pet has a favorite pillow, blanket, or bed, you must also treat the bedding since this is where fleas hide. Go easy on the herbs, since animals have a keener sense of smell than we do; too much can be overwhelming.

Under or inside the pet's pillow or cushion, place fresh or dried pennyroyal. Or sprinkle lavender essential oil directly on the bedding.

Herbal Flea Protection

fresh or dried chamomile
fresh or dried lavender
fresh or dried catnip
fresh or dried pennyroyal

Stuff a pillow with equal amounts of chamomile, lavender, and catnip. Then add double that amount with pennyroyal. Cats go wild for this.

Intestinal Worms & Parasites

Worm Remedy #1

1 tansy leaf
1 drop thyme essential oil

To rid your pet of worms, add the tansy leaf and thyme essential oil to the animal's food.

Worm Remedy #2

½ cup milk
1 teaspoon dried lavender cotton

Bring the milk to a boil. Add the lavender cotton (*Santolina chamaecyparissus*). Remove from heat, let cool, and strain. To worm your pet, old-timers recommend that the animal fast for 24 hours. Then have your cat or dog drink this milk. Cats especially find this easy to take.

Worm Remedy #3

4 tablespoons dried pumpkin seeds
½ cup boiling water

Pour boiling water over the pumpkin seeds and let them soften. Then mash the water and seeds into a creamy paste. Mix this with the animal's food.

Three hours later, dose with ¼ teaspoon castor oil. This remedy is an old-time American favorite to expel tapeworms.

Worm Remedy #4

½ cup apple-cider vinegar
1 tablespoon pau d'arco bark

Let the pau d'arco steep in the apple-cider vinegar for 2 weeks in a sunny window. Strain. Give 1 dropper per day for 3 days. Repeat in 2 weeks.

This is useful for all types of parasitic infestation.

Worm Remedy #5

1 cup apple-cider vinegar
1 teaspoon powdered black-walnut bark
1 teaspoon powdered elecampane root

Warm apple-cider vinegar on the stove. Reduce heat and add the herbs. Simmer for 5 minutes, strain, and let cool. For cats, use 1 dropper and for dogs, 2 droppers. Dose the cat or dog for 3 days. Repeat dosage after 2 weeks. This old remedy was often used to get rid of worms.

❦

Roundworm Remedy for Cats
  1 tablespoon powdered wormwood
  1 tablespoon powdered thyme
  1 tablespoon powdered garlic

Have the animal fast for 24 hours. Then mix the wormwood, thyme, and garlic. Blend well and place in #0 capsules. Give your pet 1 capsule for each 10 pounds of weight. Dose the cat four times a day. Also dose with ¼ teaspoon castor oil the first day. In 2 weeks, repeat the procedure.

Mulberry Bark Laxative

1 cup water
1 tablespoon fresh mulberry tree bark

Bring the water to a boil and add the mulberry tree bark. Boil for 10 minutes and strain. Let the animal sip the mulberry tea after it cools. This laxative kills intestinal worms.

❧

Garlic Remedies

The most common remedy for worms is garlic. It can assume the double duty of cleaning out intestinal worms and deterring fleas. Grind a clove of garlic and mix it with moist pet food. Or add garlic oil to the food; squeeze one capsule.

You can also make garlic water (see Garlic-Water Remedy, p. 302) to mix with the pet's food.

Garlic-Water Remedy

   6 cloves garlic
   2 cups water

Chop the garlic cloves and add them to the water. Bring the cloves and water to a boil; remove from heat, and cover. Let cool overnight.

   Mix 1 cup with the animal's dry food. Make sure the animal eats all the food. Next day, use the other cup of garlic water as before. Worms should be gone in a few days. Add a little garlic every day to the pet's food during flea season, and you'll have no problem with worms or fleas.

JUST FOR CATS

Cat Toys

Catnip Mice

Some cats go crazy for catnip, and you can easily grow your own plot so that your cat can have access to fresh "nip" in summer and dried "nip" in winter. It's also easy to make catnip mice for holiday treats. Simply cut out an outline of a mouse from scrap material. Stuff the mouse with cotton batting. Add a bit of dried catnip and stitch closed. Tack on some cloth or felt ears and yarn whiskers and tail.

You can make the mouse as fancy or plain as you like. You can even make a patchwork mouse, large or small, according to your cat's size and needs.

Catnip Ball

Use an old sock you don't want anymore. Fill the toe with cotton batting, using enough to make a round ball the size you want. Place some dried catnip in the ball, and tie it closed tightly with string or yarn. Make sure it won't come loose. Clip the excess sock top off, and you'll have an attractive toy that your cat will spend hours batting around. You can even leave a length of string on the ball so that you can dangle it enticingly in front of your cat.

Hint: If your cat isn't attracted to catnip, you can use powdered valerian root. Many cats find this scent very attractive.

Paper Bags

For a quick and easy toy, simply lay a few empty paper bags down on their sides and watch your pet play cat-and-mouse games.

Instead of spending all that money on pet-store scratching posts or pads, make your own. Merely save leftover carpet or old rugs. For a scratch pad, secure (staple or nail) the carpet to a square of wood. Search the hardware store to find ways to secure this square to the wall at cat height. For a scratching post, wrap the carpet around an old post or piece of wood cut to size. Nail it to a secure base, which you can also cover with this carpet.

Use a catnip spray to lead the cat to the approved scratching post or pad. Soak dried catnip in vodka for 2 weeks. Strain. Add more catnip to the liquid, and let soak again. Repeat, if necessary, until the tincture is strong enough. Place the catnip spray in a spray bottle and spritz the pad or post. You can refresh it any time.

Yarn Toy

Take a handful of yarn about 1 inch (2.5 cm) thick. Hold it in the middle and cut it so that there are 3 inches (7.5 cm) on each side. Tie the middle with a piece of yarn and leave a little yarn dangling so that you can pull the toy. Fluff. Your cat will spend hours with this toy, and you can spritz the yarn with catnip spray for added appeal. Cut the yarn ends short to make a fluffy ball or leave them long to create a limp dangler.

Surprise Box

Save your shoeboxes since they can make interesting cat toys. Simply cut different sizes and shapes in the sides and top. Insert a lightweight ball like a Ping-Pong ball or a catnip mouse. The cat will poke and prod, trying to get at the object inside.

If you use a deep box and leave the top open, the cat can hide inside.

Kitty Boutique

Shiny Fur for Cats

A cat with a good diet will have healthy-looking fur. Give your cat a bit of cottage cheese, fish leftovers, or juice from tuna or mackerel cans. You can also give your cat a dose of this tonic once in a while.

Shiny Fur Tonic
  2 cups apple-cider vinegar
  4 tablespoons cod-liver oil
  2 tablespoons powdered garlic

Mix the apple-cider vinegar, cod-liver oil, and garlic well. Add 1 teaspoon to the cat's food. Use this tonic once a month.

Cat Bed

For an easy cat bed, simply cut out two circles of fabric slightly larger than the size you want the bed. Now measure fabric for the sides. Use two long pieces of material about 4 to 6 inches (10 to 15 cm) wide—long enough to enclose the circle, but with an opening big enough to walk through.

Sew the round bottom pillow, leaving 6 inches (15 cm) open, and turn it right side out. Then sew the long side pieces together, leaving one end open, and turn it right side out. Stuff the pillow and backing with batting material. Add lavender buds to help banish fleas and to give off a pleasing scent.

Sew up the openings, and sew the back onto the pillow. Spritz the new cat bed with catnip spray if your cat is reluctant to sleep in it at first. Add stiff cardboard or plastic inserts from recycled materials to make the bottom and sides stiffer. (See p. 315.)

JUST FOR DOGS

Dog Grooming

Problem-Skin Dog Shampoo

  1 tablespoon slivered castile soap
  handful rolled oats
  2 to 4 drops tea-tree essential oil
  2 teaspoons dried chamomile

Place the slivered castile soap on a piece of muslin the size you want for a bath bag. Add the rolled oats, tea-tree essential oil, and dried chamomile. Tie this up with string or twine.

  Place the dog in a warm bath, and soap down with this bath bag. Rinse. It will make a difference if your dog has problem skin. This shampoo will soothe dry, irritated skin.

Dry Dog Shampoo

  2 cups orrisroot or cornstarch
  1 cup powdered peppermint
  1 cup powdered lavender buds

Mix the peppermint, lavender, and orris-root or cornstarch well. Store the dry shampoo in a closed container. Sprinkle it on the animal and brush in well.

Mint Dog Shampoo

  mild shampoo
  2 teaspoons peppermint
  ½ cup boiling water

Use a mild shampoo base, and mix equal amounts of strong mint tea with it. Mint is a good conditioner and scalp stimulant. It is also helpful for dandruff conditions. It has a clean, refreshing scent.

Enriching Dog Shampoo

  4 tablespoons dried soapwort
  4 teaspoons borax
  2 tablespoons dried rosemary
  5 cups boiling water

Pour boiling water over the soapwort, borax, and rosemary. Cover the mixture and let it steep for 3 days. Strain.

  Use this shampoo to enhance and condition your dog's coat. Rosemary gives a nice, clean pine scent.

For a shiny coat, make sure that your pet has a good diet. Here are some nutrition boosters that will help.

Raw Egg: For a shiny coat, try adding a raw egg to your dog's diet twice a week.

Goldenseal: Sprinkle powdered goldenseal into the dog's food. It conditions the skin and hair. Or make a tea of goldenseal, and use it as a final rinse after you shampoo the dog. Unlike raw egg, use goldenseal only when needed on rare occasions (every few months) in the dog's food. Just once or twice, at most, should suffice.

Bee Pollen: Add a little bee pollen to the dog's food.

Garlic & Brewer's Yeast: You can also add a little garlic and brewer's yeast to your pet's diet, too.

Dog Clothier

Easy-to-Make Dog Sweater

Use old sweaters that you don't want anymore. Or buy an old sweater at a yard sale;
you can get them for next to nothing. Make
this sweater as a holiday gift for your four-
legged friend or as a present for the animal
lover on your list.

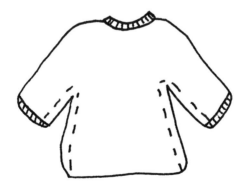

Dog Sweater

Try to find a sweater that's roughly the size of your dog. Choose a small, medium, or large in an adult or child's size.

Cut the sweater up the sides, splitting the sleeves. Measure your dog, cutting off the excess material from the body of the sweater as well as from the sleeves. Hem the bottom and sleeves, sew up the seams, and you have an instant sweater! You can spray it with stain repellant to help combat stains.

Dog Bed

Measure your dog and cut out cloth circles to make a pillow. Also cut out a long strip or tube to be used as backing.

Stuff the pillow and back it with cotton batting. Be sure you have plenty of stuffing so that the bed will be comfortable. Dogs are usually heavier than cats. Add some cedar chips to the stuffing to banish fleas and to give the bed a pleasant scent. Sew the pillow closed and sew on the backing. Make sure that you leave enough room for the dog to enter the bed. See the drawing below.

Also make sure the back is tall enough to keep out drafts and make the dog feel secure. Your pet will love it.

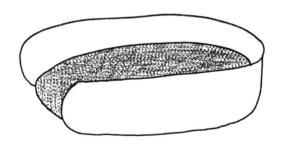

Finished Cat or Dog Bed

REMEDIES FOR BIRDS

Stomach Ailments & Diarrhea

Sometimes your canary or parakeet will develop diarrhea. This can be easily treated if you prepare a tea of caraway or fennel seeds.

Bird Diarrhea Remedy
   2 teaspoons caraway or fennel seeds
   ½ cup boiling water
   sugar cubes

Crush the caraway or fennel seeds and add them to ½ cup of boiling water. Cover and steep until cool. Strain. With a dropper, place 2 to 3 drops onto a sugar cube and place it in the cage.

Aloe Vera for Constipation
aloe-vera leaf or juice

If you notice that your bird is experiencing constipation, you can introduce a leaf from the aloe-vera plant into its cage. The bird will play and chew on the leaf and ingest some of its soothing, healing gel. You can also add pure aloe-vera juice to the pet's water.

This plant is easy to grow, doesn't take much water or care, and is very useful for all skin conditions, burns, and wounds. It is also useful internally for digestive ills. Aloe vera helps heal lesions, ulcers, and inflammations of the stomach and the rest of the digestive tract.

Asthma & Respiratory Disorders

Wild birds can find their remedies from nature. Unfortunately, our caged friends aren't free to do so. That's why we must help them out.

Bird Respiratory Remedy

  1 teaspoon dried fennel
  ½ cup boiling water
  2 teaspoons cayenne pepper
  sugar cubes

Make fennel tea, using the dried fennel and boiling water. Let steep for 10 minutes. Then mix 3 tablespoons of fennel tea with 2 teaspoons of cayenne pepper. Put a few drops on a sugar cube and place it in the bird's cage.

❦

Easy Asthma Treatments for Birds

Plantain: Become familiar with the plantain plant. Pick the plant (especially when it goes to seed) and place a sprig in the cage. This plant, easily found in most locales, is especially suited to treating a bird with asthma or breathing difficulties.

Endive & Watercress: Place fresh endive or watercress in the bird's cage for breathing difficulties. The bird will eat the amount needed.

Red Pepper: Soak a small piece of bread in milk and sprinkle it with red pepper. Place the soaked bread on a small saucer inside the cage. Don't leave it in the cage to sour.

Other Disorders

Anti-Itch Bird Spray

   4 cups distilled water
   1 teaspoon peppermint
   1 teaspoon lavender buds
   1 teaspoon rose petals
   4 to 8 drops tea-tree essential oil
   1 cup aloe-vera juice

Add the peppermint, lavender buds, and rose petals to the distilled water and bring to a boil. Remove from heat and allow the mixture to cool. Strain. Add the tea-tree essential oil to the liquid. Then mix in the aloe-vera juice.

Pour this solution into a spray bottle. Keep it at room temperature and mist the inflamed areas or the body of the bird.

Bird Immune Stimulant

1 teaspoon dandelion root
1 teaspoon burdock root
4 cups distilled water
1 teaspoon milk thistle
1 teaspoon red clover
1 to 2 cups aloe-vera juice
water

Put the dandelion and burdock roots in the distilled water and bring the herbs and water to a boil. Boil for 10 minutes. Remove from heat and add milk thistle and red clover. Cover and let it steep until cool. Strain well.

Measure and add an equal amount of aloe-vera juice. Blend.

Add half a dropper to the bird's drinking water. For large birds, you can use a full dropper. This tonic helps build up sickly birds. Dose until you notice improvement, but dose only occasionally as a tonic for healthy birds.

Mites & Scaley Leg

The bird's legs may look dry and sometimes swell. This condition is thought to be caused by mites.

Kerosene Treatment for Mites

kerosene
water

Mix equal amounts of kerosene and water. Dab small amounts onto the leg. Too much can burn or cause blistering, so be very careful. Mites are tough to get rid of and kerosene is very effective in smothering and killing them.

Rosemary Treatment for Mites

4 drops rosemary essential oil
2 tablespoons water

Add rosemary essential oil to the water.
Use this as a spray once a day to coat the
bird's legs to get rid of mites.

❧

Lice Treatment for Birds

When you introduce a new bird to your
home, sometimes the bird may be contami-
nated with lice. Place a small saucer of
water in the bottom of the cage and add 1
drop of lavender essential oil.

A bird's skin problems can result in red,
inflamed skin and feather loss.

Bird's Voice Loss

Your canary, parakeet, or parrot may some-times seem to have trouble with its voice. Try these easy remedies.

Bread & Yolk Paste: Make a paste of bread, lettuce, and rapeseed mixed with a little yolk of raw egg.

Whiskey Tonic: Apply several drops of whiskey with a pinch of sugar to the bird's drinking water. You can also use this tonic once a month as a preventative.

Feather Loss

You can try these remedies when feather loss isn't connected to moulting.

Brown Sugar: Add a bit of brown sugar to the bird's drinking water.

Cornmeal: Add some cornmeal to the bird's regular food.

Rusty Nail: You can also place a rusty (iron) nail in its drinking water along with a pinch of saffron. Ask for iron nails at the hardware store to be sure you are not getting an alloy or another metal.

Canary Feathers' Coloring

 2 tablespoons sugar
 2 tablespoons cayenne pepper
 2 tablespoons turmeric

Mix the sugar, cayenne pepper, and tumeric. Add 1 teaspoon of this mixture to the bird's daily food ration. It helps bring out the color of the canary's feathers and keeps it healthy.

❦

Egg-Laying Hints

Sometimes it takes a little coaxing to get birds in the mood for setting eggs. Hook a tea strainer inside the cage for canaries and parakeets will need a nest box.

A pinch of ground hamburger on the bottom of the cage may do the trick, but you'll have to remove any leftover meat at the end of the day.

Egg-Laying Remedy

   1 tablespoon red pepper
   2 tablespoons allspice
   4 tablespoons ginger

Mix the red pepper, allspice, and powdered ginger. Sprinkle a little on the birds' food twice a week.

Cage Care

Cleanse and disinfect cages regularly. In households with multiple birds, it is important to do this weekly and to disinfect food and water bowls, too. To disinfect, let the bowls soak in bleach water; use 2 tablespoons of bleach per gallon (3.8 liters) of hot water. Rinse and wash with hot soapy water, then dry.

For the cage, remove the bird and place some bleach water (see above) into a spray bottle. This will disinfect it perfectly; then let the cage air dry. Scrub perches with a wire brush and replace them once a year.

Thyme Wash for Bird Toys
  20 drops thyme essential oil
  2 cups water

Toys should be regularly disinfected each week. You can use thyme essential oil mixed with hot water. Rinse the toys completely and let them dry. This helps keep disease away and will keep your bird healthy and happy.

Bleach Water for Bird Toys

You can also clean bird toys with a 10% solution of bleach water. Use 2 tablespoons bleach per gallon (3.8 liters) of hot water.

Cinnamon Birdcage Cleanser

   3 tablespoons ground cinnamon
   2 cups boiling water

Make a strong tea of cinnamon with
ground cinnamon and boiling water. Steep
until cool. Strain and use to wash the
entire cage. It acts as an antiseptic.

Pest Control for Birds

Sulfur Bag

   powdered sulfur

Here's how you can keep away insects from
your birdcage. Hang a small bag of powdered sulfur at the top, outside part of the
cage, where the bird cannot get at it. This
should chase away annoying pests.

BIRD TOYS

Be careful with what you give your birds to play with. Make sure that the item is bird-safe and nonpoisonous.

❦

Toys for Large Birds

Large birds like parrots love to play and are very curious. Here's something that will keep them busy and happy.

Bottle with Beads: Fill a small clean, empty plastic soda-pop bottle with beads or other colorful objects. Replace the cap tightly. The bird will have a ball trying to get at the little treasures inside, and the bottle will make an amusing sound for its trouble.

Plastic Rings: Make a chain of plastic shower-curtain rings. String them securely to make interesting walkways. Birds seem to find this quite amusing.

Peanut-Butter Pinecone Toy

pinecone
peanut butter
birdseed

Dip a pinecone in boiling water to kill
insects and disinfect it. Let the pinecone
dry. Now smear it in peanut butter and roll
it in the birdseed.

Tie the pinecone with a piece of yarn to
the top of the cage and let it dangle. The
bird will love to eat the treats, and underneath is the toy—a pinecone to chew and
play with.

Substitution: You can substitute honey
for the peanut butter, depending on your
bird's likes or dislikes.

Tasty Ropes

   uncooked pasta or cereal "O's"
   yarn or string

Here's an easy idea to keep your bird
amused. Use yarn to string interesting
shapes of uncooked pasta. Your bird will
spend hours pushing the pasta up and
down on the string as well as chewing on
it. Colored pasta is fine.

   For another tasty treat, string a colorful
cereal shaped like little "O's" onto string or
yarn. It's really the same idea.

HOMEMADE GOODIES FOR PETS

Dog Treats

Hush Puppies

1¼ cup flour
1 cup yellow cornmeal
4½ teaspoons baking powder
1 teaspoon salt
2 tablespoons sugar
1 egg
2 cups milk
¼ cup melted shortening

Mix the flour, cornmeal, baking powder, salt, and sugar. Add the egg, milk, and melted shortening and mix well. Pour the batter onto a hot, slightly greased skillet, making tiny pancakes. Brown on both sides.

Stack and freeze these hush puppies in

small amounts so that you can thaw them out for occasional treats—to hush your own puppy.

Mush Cakes

  1 pound (454 g) chicken neck bones
  garlic cloves
  cornmeal
  water

Place the neck bones in a large pan of boiling water. Add several cloves of garlic and boil until the meat is tender. Pick the meat off the bones. Discard the bones. Return the broth to the stove and boil, slowly adding cornmeal and sifting it through the fingers as you stir constantly. Keep adding cornmeal until the mixture is very thick. Turn the heat to the lowest possible setting and cook 45 minutes, stirring occasionally.

Rinse a flat cake pan with cold water (this prevents sticking), and pour the mixture into the cake pan. Place the mush cake(s) in the refrigerator to cool. Slice the mush cake and serve it cold to your pet. You can use this instead of regular food or as a treat. It keeps a week in the refrigerator.

If you slice and fry it, serving it with maple syrup, the whole family can eat it. It's great!

Begging Strips

2 cups rye flour
1 cup cornmeal
2 cups chopped ham
2 tablespoons desiccated liver
4 tablespoons bonemeal
2 to 4 eggs
½ cup bacon fat
water

Mix the flour, cornmeal, ham, liver, bonemeal, eggs, and bacon fat. Add enough water to form a stiff dough. Roll out the dough and cut it into strips.

Bake the strips in a low oven at 300° F (149° C). Bake until they are dry to touch.

Meatloaf Special

2 cups cooked rice
½ cup hamburger
½ cup pork and beans
½ cup shredded carrots
1 tablespoon wheat germ
½ to 1 cup crushed crackers
2 to 3 eggs

Mix the cooked rice, hamburger, pork and beans, carrots, wheat germ, and crushed crackers. Add enough eggs so that the mixture holds together. Bake in the oven at 300° F (149° C) until browned. Slice and freeze.

For a treat, give your pet small slices.

Tasty Chicken-Liver Biscuits

  1 pound (454 g) cooked chicken livers
  2 cups whole-wheat flour
  1 cup cornmeal
  1 to 2 eggs

Crumble the cooked chicken livers and add the flour, cornmeal, and eggs. The mixture should be a doughy consistency; add water if it is too dry. Spread the dough in a pan and score it into squares. Bake at 325° F (163° C) for 20 to 25 minutes. Turn the oven off and let the biscuits cool in the oven.

  Break the biscuits apart and store them in a closed container in the refrigerator.

Wheaty Dog Snacks

1½ cups whole-wheat flour
4 tablespoons bacon grease
½ cup chicken stock
1 teaspoon bonemeal

Mix the flour, bacon grease, chicken stock, and bonemeal well. Roll out very thin, about the thickness of a cracker, on a cookie sheet. Cut the dough into rectangles. Bake until golden brown at 350° F (177° C) for 15 to 20 minutes. Break the cracker snacks apart when cooled.

Store them in a tightly closed container.

Dog Cookies

    3 cups whole-wheat flour
    2 cups oatmeal
    ¼ cup wheat germ
    ¼ cup dry milk
    1 ⅓ cups water
    2 minced garlic cloves
    ⅓ cup peanut butter
    1 egg

Mix the flour, oatmeal, wheat germ, and dry milk. Add the water, garlic cloves, peanut butter, and egg. Mix well. Roll out the dough and cut it into shapes with a cookie cutter.

Put these cookie shapes on a greased cookie sheet. Bake at 300° F (149° C) for 1 hour 45 minutes.

To keep them fresh, store the dog cookies in airtight containers.

Ultra Dog Biscuits

2½ cups flour
¼ cup sunflower seeds
¼ cup cornmeal
2 tablespoons olive oil
¼ cup molasses or honey
¼ cup milk
2 eggs
1 teaspoon salt

Mix the flour, sunflower seeds, and cornmeal. Add the olive oil, molasses or honey, milk, eggs, and salt. Mix well. Knead into a firm dough. Roll out and cut into strips 4 inches (10 cm) long. Twist two strips together and lay them out on cookie sheets. Bake at 350° F (177° C) for 30 minutes. Turn off the oven and let them cool in the oven.

Store the biscuits in a closed container.

Cheesy Dog Biscuits

2½ cups flour
¼ cup dry milk
1 cup bulgur
1 cup chicken broth
½ cup cornmeal
¼ cup parsley
1¼ cups shredded cheddar cheese
water as needed
1 egg
1 tablespoon milk

Blend the flour, dry milk, and bulgar. Add the chicken broth. Then stir in the cornmeal, parsley, and cheddar cheese to make a stiff dough. Add a little warm water if necessary to work it better. On a floured surface, roll out the dough to ¼ inch thick. Cut with a cookie cutter into desired shapes. Transfer the cut dough to cookie sheets.

Beat 1 egg with 1 tablespoon of milk and use to glaze the biscuits. Bake at 300° F (149° C) for 20 minutes. Turn off the oven. Let the biscuits sit in the oven overnight. Store them in closed containers.

Cat Treats

Kitty Krunchies

1 can mackerel
2 teaspoons salt
2 cups flour
2 tablespoons bacon grease
2 teaspoons cod-liver oil
1 cup cornmeal
2 cloves minced garlic
½ cup wheat germ
1 capsule or ⅛ teaspoon vitamin E oil
½ cup dry milk
2 cups water
¼ cup nutritional yeast

Mix the mackerel, salt, flour, bacon grease, cod-liver oil, cornmeal, minced garlic, wheat germ, and vitamin E oil. Add the dry milk and water and blend. Roll out the dough and cut it into little bits.

Bake at 350° F (177° C) for 40 minutes. Sprinkle the treats with the yeast and cool. Store them in airtight containers.

Dried Liver Strips
  calf liver
  garlic powder

Rinse calf liver and boil it until tender. Cool. Slice in strips and place in a food dehydrator or low oven. Sprinkle with garlic powder. Dry until leathery.

Store in an airtight container.

Potato Crisps

   1 cup mashed potatoes
   2 tablespoons grated carrots
   ½ cup cottage cheese
   ¼ cup grated cheddar cheese
   1 cup flour
   1 egg

Blend the mashed potatoes, carrots, cottage cheese, and cheddar cheese. Add the flour and egg. Mix well. Make a thick paste. Place small dollops on greased cookie sheets. Bake in a low oven until brown and crisp. Cool.

   Store these potato crisps in the refrigerator in a closed container.

Wild Bird Treats

Around the holidays, the family can enjoy making special treats for wild birds and watching them eat the tasty morsels.

Bird Treat Balls

3½ cups rolled oats
4 cups water
2 cups lard
1½ cups crunchy peanut butter
3½ cups cornmeal
3½ cups creamy wheat cereal

Cook the rolled oats in water for two minutes. Stir in the lard, peanut butter, cornmeal, and cereal until well blended. Cool and shape into balls. Put these treat balls in mesh bags and decorate them with ribbon to hang. Cream of Wheat works well in this recipe.

Bird Cookies

1 cup cornmeal
1 cup flour
1 cup bread crumbs
½ tablespoon baking soda
¾ cup raisins
½ cup bacon grease
1 cup water
cooking-oil spray
string

Combine the cornmeal, flour, bread crumbs, baking soda, raisins, bacon grease, and water. Mix well.

Spray cookie sheets with cooking oil. Lay out string in loops. Drop by teaspoonfuls onto the loops of string so that each cookie will have a baked-in hanger. Bake 350° F (177° C) for 15 minutes. Cool. Attach these bird cookies to tree branches.

Pinecone Treats

pinecones
peanut butter
birdseed
raisins or cereal
ribbon or fishing line

Collect pinecones. Roll them in peanut butter. Mix birdseed with raisins or cereal. Roll the pinecones in this mix. Attach ribbon or fishing line to the pinecones.

Hang them outside to feed and tempt birds within view of your windows.

Birdseed Cakes

2 cups birdseed
5 cups cracked corn
1 cup peanut butter
1 cup melted suet
string

Mix the birdseed, cracked corn, peanut butter, and melted suet well. Grease a muffin tin. Lay looped string across each muffin-tin hole, spooning this mixture over the string, so that you have little cakes with string hangers. Let the cakes cool so that the suet again becomes solid. (Do not bake.)

Hang the birdseed cakes on tree branches as treats.

Suet Squares

suet
birdseed

You can easily make suet squares for your suet feeders. It will cost only pennies. Ask the butcher or someone at the grocery meat counter for some suet. Melt the suet in a pan and remove from heat. Mix in birdseed. Line cake pans with waxed paper. Pour in the mixture and let cool. When cool, slice the suet and birdseed into squares to fit your bird feeder. Keep cool.

Wild Bird Mix

2 pounds (1 kg) cornmeal
2 pounds (1 kg) pea meal
2 pounds (1 kg) thistle seeds
2 pounds (1 kg) cracked corn
2 pounds (1 kg) bread crumbs
2 pounds (1 kg) millet seeds
2 pounds (1 kg) sunflower seeds
¾ cup (6 ounces or 200 g) cayenne pepper
1 pound (500 g) suet or lard

Melt the lard and pour it over the cornmeal, pea meal, thistle seeds, cracked corn, bread crumbs, millet seeds, sunflower seeds, and cayenne pepper. Mix the seeds thoroughly. This seed mixture will attract all kinds of bird species.

The metric equivalents have been rounded off and adjusted for shopping convenience.

Redbird Feed

1 pound (500 g) sunflower seeds
1 pound (500 g) cracked wheat
2 pounds (1 kg) Canary Feed (recipe, p. 354)

Mix the sunflower seeds, cracked wheat, and Canary Feed well. Grind it into a coarse powder.

Dove Feed

4 pounds (2 kg) red and yellow millet seeds
1 pound (500 g) buckwheat
1 pound (500 g) crushed wheat
½ pound (250 g) cracked corn
¼ cup uncooked rice
¼ cup cracked dried peas

Mix the millet seeds, buckwheat, crushed wheat, cracked corn, rice, and dried peas well. Provide feed daily and your local doves will soon become regulars.

Mockingbird Feed

1 pound (500 g) poppy seeds
1 pound (500 g) cornmeal
1 pound (500 g) pea meal
¼ cup uncooked rice
1 pound (500 g) cracked corn
1 tablespoon cayenne pepper
lard
dried, grated carrots (optional)

Grind the poppy seeds, cornmeal, pea meal, rice, and cracked corn. Add the cayenne pepper and pour a little lard over the mix, just for flavor. Add dried, grated carrots in equal amounts, if you choose.

Mockingbirds and other wild birds will love this.

Domestic Bird Feed & Treats

Why mix your own feed? You can purchase quality feed that has not been sprayed with chemicals or had anything added to it that you don't know about. Unadulterated feed makes a healthier, stronger bird.

Canary Feed

2 tablespoons poppy seeds
2 tablespoons powdered cuttlefish
4 tablespoons dried, powdered egg yolk
4 tablespoons granulated sugar
1 cup crushed wheat crackers

Mix the poppy seeds, powdered cuttlefish, dried egg yolk, sugar, and wheat crackers well. Feed your bird daily.

Sweet Mix for Canaries & Parakeets

½ pound (250 g) brown sugar
1 pound (500 g) ground pea meal
4 tablespoons fresh butter
2 hard-cooked egg yolks
¼ cup poppy seeds
¼ cup thistle seeds

Mix the brown sugar, pea meal, butter, and hard-cooked egg yolks well. Brown in a frying pan. Add the poppy and thistle seeds. Keep the mix refrigerated.

Parrot Feed

½ pound (250 g) sunflower seeds
4 tablespoons safflower seeds
2 tablespoons millet seeds
2 tablespoons ground nuts, any kind
2 tablespoons buckwheat
1 tablespoon cayenne pepper

Mix the sunflower seeds, safflower seeds, millet seeds, nuts, buckwheat, and cayenne pepper well. Parrots go crazy for this.

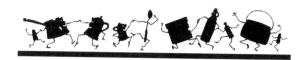

Part 4
HOUSE & GARDEN

Many helpful house and garden products can be homemade. You'll find recipes for furniture wax and polish for silver, brass, and copper. Find an easy way to polish shoes and waterproof boots.

You can make your own cleaning supplies, sprays, disinfectants, and washes for kitchen and bath. Here are quick ways to clean drains, toilet bowls, carpets, and windows.

If you have mold, mildew, odors, or pests, like rats or mice, in your basement or food storage rooms, use the easy remedies. You can also get rid of flies and other pests around garbage cans.

Insect repellants for the house that get rid of fleas, mosquitoes, moths, bees, roaches, and ants are practical and effective. Easy plant and garden sprays include natural fertilizers, weed killers, and natural insecticides. You find hints for ridding outdoor plants of worms and other invaders.

For the laundry, you'll find spot and stain removers, homemade starch, and ways to clean old lace and tablecloths.

Indulge in soapmaking and candlemaking, whether plain or fancy. Create your own dry or moist potpourri, pomanders, rose beads, scent bags, room sprays, air fresheners, and room deodorants.

FURNITURE WAX

Here are some furniture waxes or polishes to keep your wooden furniture clean and shiny. It's best to dust furniture before applying the wax or polish. Some polish may be more suitable for dark rather than light wood finishes.

Fine Furniture Wax

- 1 cup linseed oil
- 1 cup beer
- 2 tablespoons hydrochloric acid (muriatic acid)
- 2 tablespoons rubbing alcohol
- 1 beaten egg white

Beat the egg white until foamy. Mix the linseed oil, beer, hydrochloric acid, alcohol, and egg white well. Keep the wax in a sealed bottle.

Dust the furniture and apply this wax with a soft flannel cloth. Polish with a silk handkerchief.

Almond Furniture Polish

rubbing alcohol
white vinegar
sweet almond oil

Use equal parts of alcohol and white vinegar. Then add sweet almond oil, using just a little more than the amount of alcohol. Shake the bottle well each day for 3 weeks; the longer it sets, the better it will be.

To use, apply this polish to the furniture and rub until dry. Apply to furniture every three months. For a dining table you use every day, you can polish it each week. This polish gives a brilliant shine.

Best Wood Polish

  2 tablespoons melted beeswax
  1 cup turpentine

Blend the melted beeswax and turpentine well. Apply lightly with a soft cloth. Buff to a shine with a clean rag.

Caution: Don't use this polish on painted furniture; it will act as a paint remover.

Easy Furniture Polish

  1 cup olive oil or vegetable oil
  1 cup white vinegar

Mix the olive oil and vinegar and bring to a boil. Boil for 10 minutes. Let cool and bottle. To use, dip a cloth in the mixture and buff the furniture well.

Lemon-Bright Furniture Polish

  2 teaspoons olive oil
  2 teaspoons lemon juice
  2 teaspoons whiskey
  2 teaspoons water

Mix the olive oil, lemon juice, whiskey, and water well. Rub into the wood; then buff for a deep shine.

❧

Unwaxed Wood Polish

  ½ cup vegetable oil
  ½ cup lemon juice

Mix the vegetable oil and lemon juice well. Apply a thin coat to the furniture to make the wood gleam.

If you apply this polish evenly, it can be used on unstained or untreated wood.

Dark Furniture Scratch Cover

  2 teaspoons instant coffee
  4 teaspoons water

Mix the instant coffee and water into a thick paste. Apply it to the scratch with a cotton ball. Let sit 5 minutes and wipe off.

  You can also make a paste with water and black-walnut hulls.

  This works on dark wooden furniture.

Light Furniture Scratch Cover

  lemon oil

Use lemon oil to hide scratches on light-colored wooden furniture, like beech or birch.

Dark Furniture Stain

strong black tea

Make a strong black tea and let cool. Use as a wash over the wood. This brings out the wood grain and darkens the wood.

❧

Remover for White Rings

table salt
shortening

Sometimes wooden furniture will develop white rings when hot plates or cups are set on them. Here's a remedy.

Sprinkle salt over the white marks. Dip a clean cloth in the shortening and rub the salt into the rings. If the discoloration isn't too deep, this should take out the marks.

SILVER, BRASS & COPPER POLISH

Silver & Stainless Steel

Stainless-Steel Sink Polish

  olive oil

To make stainless-steel sinks shine, clean them well and then polish with olive oil. Wipe dry.

Traditional Silver Cleaners

These silver cleaners, meant for silver utensils and jewelry, also work well on stainless-steel fixtures such as those in the kitchen or bathroom. Do not soak silver objects longer than the recommended time (20 minutes) in a solution or paste.

Baking-Soda Paste: Make a simple paste of baking soda and water. Scrub and rinse the silver.

Silver Soak: Soak silver jewelry or silver utensils in warm water to which 1 teaspoon of baking soda, 1 teaspoon of salt, and a piece of aluminum foil have been added. Soak 20 minutes then wipe dry with a soft cloth.

Toothpaste: You can also rub the tarnished piece with toothpaste (not the gel kind). Rinse and polish dry.

Wood-Ash Paste: An old remedy calls for mixing wood ashes with water to form a paste that will make the tarnish disappear.

Copper & Brass

Brass Polish

    4 tablespoons flour
    4 tablespoons salt
    2 tablespoons water or white vinegar

Mix the flour, salt, and water into a thick paste. Add more water if the mixture is too dry. Rub onto brass with a soft cloth. Rinse; then polish dry. Or mix equal parts of salt and flour with a little white vinegar and rub.

Copper & Brass Cleaner

1 cup warm water
1 cup flour
1 cup salt
1 cup powdered detergent
1¼ cups white vinegar
½ cup lemon juice

Mix the water, flour, salt, detergent, white vinegar, and lemon juice well in a plastic bucket. Store the cleaner in a half-gallon (2-liter) jug. To use, shake well, apply to cookware, and polish. Rinse and buff with a dry cloth.

Easy Copper & Brass Polishes

Here are other easy, traditional ways to polish the copper and brass in your house.

Buttermilk: Rub the copper or brass object with hot buttermilk.

Lemon, Salt & Vinegar: Use a cut lemon and dip it in a solution of equal parts of salt and vinegar. Rub down and buff dry.

Salt, Vinegar & Flour Paste: Make a paste with equal parts salt and vinegar with flour. Coat the object and let it sit a few minutes. Rinse and dry.

Ketchup Polish: For brass, use ketchup. Pour it on the object to be cleaned and let it sit for 10 minutes. Then rinse and wipe dry.

SHOE POLISH & WATERPROOFING

Lemon Shoe Polish

fresh lemon

Cut a lemon in half. Use half to rub all over one leather boot or shoe. Buff just as you would with regular shoe polish. Use the other lemon half to polish the other shoe.

Boot & Shoe Waterproofing

beeswax
lanolin

You can waterproof leather boots and shoes by warming equal amounts of beeswax and lanolin until melted and well mixed. Use a cloth to apply this all over the top and bottom of the boots, taking care to remember the stitched areas. Buff the boots as needed.

JEWELRY POLISH

For cleaning and polishing jewelry, also consult the brass, copper, and silver cleaners, depending on the type of jewelry. Of course, gold jewelry doesn't require polish. But artificial gold, made from metal alloys, may come clean in lemon juice concentrate. Or simply wipe off the green film.

Silver Jewelry Cleaner
   lemon juice concentrate

Soak the silver jewelry in lemon-juice concentrate for 20 minutes. Rinse well and buff dry. The tarnish should wipe off quite easily.

CLEANING SUPPLIES

Your kitchen cupboard probably has most ingredients for these cleaning supplies. You can make your own cleaning supplies inexpensively without the harsh chemicals, perfumes, and dyes found in many commercial products. You can also avoid the headaches and allergies you may get when using them. The best commercial products usually contain one or more of the basic ingredients used in these homemade recipes.

Lemon juice kills bacteria on surfaces it touches. Cloves and marjoram help disinfect. Baking soda absorbs odors and helps everything smell fresh. Ammonia or vinegar are great for cleaning glass and mirrors. Just avoid cleansers and abrasives, like alcohol or hydrogen peroxide, on plastics. They may become cloudy. Use soap and water for clear plastic bathroom glasses and soap trays.

Caution: Never combine bleach and ammonia since together they create dangerous fumes.

ॐ

All-Purpose Cleaning Sprays & Washes

Baking Soda Wash
  1 gallon (3.8 liters) warm water
  1 cup baking soda

Mix the warm water and baking soda well. Store this cleaner in a spray bottle to keep handy. Or mix it up to use when mopping the floor.

  This cleaner is useful for washing windows, cleaning compact discs, mopping vinyl floors, and more.

Everyday Cleaning Spray

¼ cup ammonia
2 tablespoons apple-cider vinegar
1 tablespoon baking soda
½ gallon (1.8 liters) water

Mix the ammonia, apple-cider vinegar, baking soda, and water. Pour some in a handy spray bottle. Use the spray to clean counters, walls, tubs, sinks, and showers.

❧

Cinnamon Cleaning Spray

1 tablespoon dried elder flowers
1 cup boiling water
25 drops cinnamon essential oil

Make a strong elder-flower tea, using the dried elder flowers and boiling water. Add 25 drops cinnamon essential oil per cup. Pour the solution into a spray bottle.

This is good for cleaning the modern-day refrigerator; it leaves a nice, fresh scent. You can also spray it around the basement to kill mold. This makes musty smells disappear. Elder flower discourages molds and fungi, and cinnamon essential oil kills molds and germs.

❦

Kitchen & Bath

Tile & Grout Scrub

⅔ cup ammonia
½ cup white vinegar
1 cup baking soda
1 gallon (3.8 liters) warm water

Mix the ammonia, white vinegar, baking soda, and warm water in a bucket. Pour into gallon (4-liter) glass jar to store. Use a spray bottle to spray and wipe tile.

Homemade Scouring Powder

soap, bar or liquid
table salt, baking soda, or borax

Soap up a scrub brush and sprinkle table
salt, baking soda, or borax on the bristles
to deep clean.

Mildew Cleanser

½ cup liquid soap
½ cup baking soda
1 gallon (3.8 liters) vinegar

Mix the liquid soap, baking soda, and
vinegar. Use the solution to sponge down
bathroom tiles. Add this to the washing
machine to cleanse a mildew-covered
shower curtain.

For other uses, add ¼ cup of this cleanser
to 2 quarts (1.9 liters) warm water and mix

well. This disinfects and cleans well.

Bleach, though perhaps harsher, when added to the washing machine also rids a shower curtain of mildew.

Marjoram Kitchen Disinfectant

  4 cups boiling water
  4 cups fresh sweet marjoram
  1 tablespoon whole cloves
  1 tablespoon lemon juice
  1 tablespoon mild liquid soap

Pour the boiling water over the marjoram and cloves. Let cool and strain. Add the lemon juice and mild liquid soap. Mix well and pour the solution into a spray bottle. Saturate areas that you want to disinfect.

Citrus Kitchen Disinfectant Spray

3 drops eucalyptus essential oil
3 drops lemon essential oil
3 drops grapefruit essential oil
1 cup water

Mix equal amounts of eucalyptus, lemon, and grapefruit essential oils. Add 8 drops of this mixture to 1 cup of water in a spray bottle.

Spray this disinfectant on cutting boards and counters. This spray will disinfect wooden salad bowls, too.

You can also spray this on no-wax floors to disinfect the whole kitchen and leave a pleasant scent.

Baking Soda & Water: Make a solution of baking soda and water to clean the refrigerator and freezer. Keep an open box of baking soda in the refrigerator to absorb odors year-round. Replace the box the next time you clean.

White Vinegar: Use white vinegar to clean and deodorize a refrigerator or freezer.

Drains

Quick Salt Drain Cleanser
  salt
  hot water

Pour salt down the drain and flush with hot water to freshen and cleanse quickly.

Baking Soda & Vinegar Drain Cleanser

¼ cup baking soda
½ cup vinegar

Pour the baking soda down the drain; then follow with the vinegar. It will fizz up, and when the fizzing is done, you can flush the drain with hot water. This gets rid of bad drain smells and sweetens the kitchen.

Toilet Bowls

Baking Soda & Vinegar: Use the recipe for the Baking Soda & Vinegar Drain Cleanser above on this page to clean the toilet bowl. Scrub the toilet with a brush and baking soda and vinegar. Then let the mixture sit overnight to get rid of heavy stains or lime deposits.

Lemon & Rosemary Toilet-Bowl Disinfectant

   10 drops tea-tree essential oil
   10 drops lemon essential oil
   10 drops rosemary essential oil
   3 cups white vinegar

Mix the tea-tree, lemon, and rosemary essential oils. Add the white vinegar. Keep the disinfectant in a spray bottle in a dark area. Spray the toilet inside and out to cleanse, disinfect, and deodorize. This disinfectant kills even the strongest bacteria and molds.

   You can also use this disinfectant to spray down shower curtains, grout, or any area with mold.

❧

Thyme Toilet-Bowl Disinfectant

   2 cups boiling water
   2 cups dried thyme
   ½ cup powdered laundry detergent

Pour boiling water over the thyme. Steep for 10 minutes and strain. Add the laundry detergent. Pour the solution into a plastic 2-cup spray bottle. Use it to clean and disinfect toilets.

Carpets

Dry-Carpet Cleaner

   1 cup cornmeal
   ½ cup borax

Mix the cornmeal and borax. Sprinkle the cleaner on carpet stains. Let sit for 30 minutes to 1 hour. Vacuum thoroughly.

Carpet-Stain Cleaner

½ cup mild liquid soap
2 cups hot water

Whip the liquid soap and hot water to foam in a blender. Apply the foam with a sponge. Wipe clean with a cloth.

Windows

Alcohol & Vinegar Window Cleaner

2 cups rubbing alcohol
2 cups cold water
⅛ cup white vinegar

Mix the alcohol, water, and white vinegar. Pour the solution into a spray bottle to clean windows, polish appliances, and cut grease.

Easy Lemon Juice Window Cleaner

2 tablespoons lemon juice
4 cups water

Simply add lemon juice to water and wipe your windows clean.

Lemon & Vinegar Window Cleaner

1 cup white vinegar
3 cups water
20 drops lemon essential oil

Mix the white vinegar, water, and lemon essential oil. Use a clean cloth or paper towel dipped in this solution to clean windows. This makes a fresh-smelling window cleanser.

BASEMENTS & FOOD STORAGE

Mold, Mildew & Odors

Traditional Root Cellars

Before ice boxes and refrigerators, households kept milk, butter, and other goods cool in root cellars. Root cellars were good places to store potatoes, carrots, and cabbages as well as home-canned products.

Sometimes these cellars, dug into the side of a hill or sitting below the house, became musty smelling. To deter bad smells, people used bundles of sweet-smelling herbs—lavender, mint, or spices, like cloves or cinnamon, if they had them on hand.

Cinnamon & Elder Flower Cleaning Spray

1 cup boiling water
2 tablespoons elder flowers
25 drops cinnamon essential oil

Make an elder-flower tea, using 2 tablespoons elder flowers to 1 cup boiling water. Steep for 10 minutes. This strong tea discourages molds and fungi. Per cup of tea, add 25 drops cinnamon essential oil, which kills molds and germs. Pour the liquid into a spray bottle.

Spray around the basement to kill mold. This makes musty smells disappear. You can also use the spray to clean the refrigerator; it leaves a nice fresh scent.

This all-purpose spray eliminates the mess of traditional dried-herb bundles and the need to change the bundles. You can make batches of the spray when elder flowers bloom in early summer and have it on hand the rest of the year.

❦

Brimstone Disinfectant

brimstone (stick sulfur)

Getting rid of mold and mildew has long been important since many cellars were traditionally used for food storage, and mold would quickly destroy the produce. In the early 20th century, people used something called stick sulfur (brimstone).

They placed it on a pan, closed the basement or cellar tightly, and burned the sulfur. It killed the mold. They would also do this in the house if there had been a serious infectious illness to disinfect the whole household.

Disinfecting Wash

   1 box baking soda
   small pail water
   ½ teaspoon tea-tree essential oil
   ½ teaspoon eucalyptus essential oil

Mix the baking soda in the water. Add the tea-tree and eucalyptus essential oils. Wash down moldy areas. This disinfecting wash will leave a clean, pleasant scent and help rid cellars of mold and mildew.

Mice & Rats

Peppermint Chaser

   dried peppermint, peppermint essential oil,
   or peppermint tea

If rats, mice, or even spiders are a problem, you can use traditional methods to effectively banish them without resorting to poisons or expensive traps. Many old-time recipe books contained recipes with peppermint and described this easy method to make rats or mice flee homes.

In earlier centuries, ratcatchers cleared buildings by using this herb. They blocked any holes with rags soaked in peppermint oil. You could also make bags of dried peppermint to lay in corners or spray a solution of strong peppermint tea around the basement periodically.

Garbage Cans

Lavender & Thyme Garbage Can Wash
dried or fresh lavender
dried or fresh thyme
water
lavender essential oil

To keep your garbage can disinfected and sweet smelling, use equal amounts of lavender and thyme tea to make a wash. This lavender and thyme wash should discourage mold or sour smells on indoor or outdoor garbage cans.

To keep flies away, add a few extra drops of lavender essential oil to the bottom of the cans.

INSECT REPELLANTS

All-Purpose Household Insect Repellants

Camphor Insect Spray

  1 block camphor
  1 ounce (28 g) menthol crystals
  2 cups alcohol

Here's another mixture to drive away six-legged and eight-legged creepies. Shave a block of camphor into a glass bowl. Add the menthol crystals. Stir with a wooden spoon until it becomes a liquid; this will take a few minutes. Add the mixture to the alcohol.

Pour this into a spray bottle and spray crevices and places where creepy crawlies hide.

Borax Chaser

powdered borax

Borax drives away most insects. Sprinkle powdered borax around the haunts of insects to keep them away. Back corners of kitchen cupboards and near the outside edges of windowsills are good spots.

Southern homes have long favored this remedy for ridding the premises of roaches. You need to renew the borax every six months or so. Just make sure you keep pets out of the borax.

Fleas

Soapy-Water Pan: If you have a flea infestation in the house or in a particular room, pour water and a little dishwashing liquid into a shallow foil pie plate. Mix well. At night, place the pan on the floor in the middle of the room. Then turn on a small light directed over the dish.

Go to bed. In the morning, the pan will be filled with fleas, and you can pour its contents into the toilet and flush. This trick works well; during the night, fleas are attracted to the light.

Rock Salt & Pennyroyal: To banish fleas, put rock salt and dried pennyroyal in foam trays and slide them under beds, couches, or chairs.

Caution: Make sure that children cannot get into these trays and pans.

❧
Carpet Care for Flea Infestation

Here's what to do for carpets that are infested with fleas.

Boric Acid: Sprinkle carpets with boric acid to kill fleas and other pests. Let sit for 25 minutes; then vacuum.

Diatomaceous Earth: Sprinkle the carpet with diatomaceous earth. Let sit for 25 minutes. Vacuum up the fleas.

Camphor Essential Oil: Add 5 to 6 drops of camphor essential oil to a cotton ball and place it in the bag of your vacuum cleaner. It will kill fleas and eggs as you sweep them up. For this to work effectively, you must vacuum every day and refresh the cotton ball each week.

Carpet Cleaner for Fleas

   powdered rosemary
   powdered peppermint
   powdered lemongrass
   baking soda

Use equal amounts of powdered rosemary, peppermint, and lemongrass. Mix well. Then add half as much baking soda. Keep the powder in a closed container. Sprinkle sparingly on carpets. After 20 minutes, vacuum the carpet.

  This is a little like the old practice of strewing herbs around the house, without the mess, since the vacuum cleaner removes the herbs and baking soda.

Eucalyptus & Pennyroyal Flea Repellant

   1 cup white vinegar
   ½ teaspoon eucalyptus essential oil
   ½ teaspoon pennyroyal essential oil

Mix the white vinegar and the eucalyptus and pennyroyal essential oils. Pour the solution into a spray bottle. Frequently mist areas of flea infestation and along walls and doorways. This repellant has a pleasant scent that helps freshen the room.

Flea Body Spray

1 cup boiling water
1 teaspoon chamomile
1 teaspoon powdered valerian root
1 teaspoon powdered licorice root
1 teaspoon peppermint
1 cup witch hazel

Pour boiling water over the chamomile, valerian root, licorice root, and peppermint. Steep until cool. Strain. Add the witch hazel. Pour into a spray bottle. Mist arms and legs to repel fleas and other insects.

Mosquitoes & Other Pests

Basil & Lavender Mosquito Rub

½ cup rubbing alcohol
1 tablespoon basil
broken cinnamon stick
½ teaspoon lavender essential oil

Add the basil and broken cinnamon to the alcohol. Let this steep for 2 weeks and strain. Add the lavender essential oil and mix well.

Pour a small amount into the hand and rub on your arms, neck, legs. Use care on the face. This is a good mosquito deterrent. Use it when you'll be outdoors at dusk for any length of time.

Lavender Mosquito Rub

½ teaspoon lavender essential oil
4 tablespoons unscented hand lotion

Add lavender essential oil to unscented hand lotion and rub it into exposed skin. Although this may be pleasant-smelling to you, insects don't like it.

❧

Vinegar & Catnip Rub

catnip
lavender buds
spearmint
apple-cider vinegar

Fill a Mason jar with catnip, lavender buds, and spearmint. Cover the herbs with apple-cider vinegar. Steep in a sunny window for 2 weeks. Strain. Use as a body rub to repel pests.

Basil Mosquito & Fly Repellant

dried or fresh basil or basil essential oil

To get rid of flies or mosquitoes, on low heat, simmer a pan of water on the stove and add basil to the hot water. The scent repels flies and mosquitoes.

Grow basil in the windowsill or near doorways. You can also banish pests from picnics if you light a candle and add a few drops of basil essential oil to the melted wax on top. The scent will linger in the air and deter flying insects.

Vanilla Bug-Off Remedy

  2 vanilla beans
  2 cups (1 pint or 480 ml) vodka

Break the fresh vanilla beans and add them to the vodka. Let steep for 2 weeks or more. Strain. For a stronger scent, repeat the procedure. Rub onto exposed areas of the skin. Reapply as needed. Vanilla has a great smell and keeps bugs away.

Stinky Valerian Repellant

  ¼ cup powdered valerian root
  2 cups vodka

Steep the valerian root in vodka for 2 weeks. Strain. Rub on all over. Although it smells bad, you won't be bothered by biting flies, mosquitoes, or gnats. This repellant is good for camping or working in the garden and when you need heavy-duty protection.

Cedarwood Pest Oil

  ¼ cup olive oil
  10 drops tea-tree essential oil
  10 drops peppermint essential oil
  20 drops cedarwood essential oil

Mix the olive oil with the tea-tree, peppermint, and cedarwood essential oils. Pour the oil into a spray bottle and mist the skin. Keep out of eyes or sensitive areas.

Moths

Lavender Moth Repellant

  dried lavender buds
  fresh unbudded lavender stems
  lemon and orange peels

Wrap up little bundles of dried lavender buds with orange and lemon peels in a mesh bag, tie them with a ribbon, and hang them in the closet to keep moths away from sweaters and important, stored clothing.

🍃

You can also make a lavender wand by picking about 15 stems of lavender that have not quite budded out yet. Tie them just under the buds with ribbon. Then fold 9 of the stems down over the lavender buds, tying above the buds, and weave a ribbon through the stems, tying a pretty bow below the "encased" buds. Trim stems at the bottom evenly and tie a ribbon at the very end from which you can hang the lavender wand. Dry for 1 week.

Hang or place these lavender sprays in a drawer with clothing and they will chase away moths and give the clothing a pleasing scent.

Citrus Moth Repellant

lemon or orange peel

Moths hate the smell of citrus fruits and peels. Make up bags of dried lemon or orange peels to tuck among your fine clothing. This is an old remedy.

Bees & Spiders

Bee-Sting & Spider-Bite Remedies

These bee-sting remedies are also good for spider bites.

Basil: If you get stung by a bee, be sure to have fresh basil growing in your yard. Rub a leaf over the bee sting; it will take away both the pain and the swelling.

Lavender: Lavender essential oil also relieves the pain and swelling of a bee sting or spider bite.

Roaches

Hot Alum Water

½ cup alum
4 cups boiling water

Add the alum to the boiling water. While hot, use a paintbrush to apply it to cracks and other places bugs are found. This kills ants, roaches, spiders, or any creepy crawler.

Molasses Pot

molasses or honey
cooking pot

Coat the insides of an old soup pot with honey or molasses. Put the pot against a wall where you see roaches. Leave overnight. In the morning, the pot will be licked clean and you'll find roaches in the bottom of the pot. Pour boiling water over them.

Boric Acid

borax or boric acid

Sprinkle powdered boric acid or borax under the kitchen sink, in the corners of cupboards, and in crevices or cracks where bugs might hide. This method works quite well. It is popular in Texas and the South for ridding house of roaches. You'll need to refresh the boric acid every 6 months. Although this is less toxic than use of insect sprays, you'll want to keep pets out of the boric acid.

Sticky Paper

6 ounces (168 g) rosin
1 tablespoon melted shortening

To catch ants, flies, and roaches, use an old pot or pan bought at a yard sale. Melt the rosin with the shortening. It should form a very thick mixture. Spread with an old knife or stick onto cardboard. Place this where pets and children cannot reach. Pests will stick to it and when it's filled, you can toss in the trash.

Ants

Homemade Ant Killer
⅓ cup white vinegar
3 tablespoons lemon-scented dishwashing liquid
⅔ cup water

Mix the vinegar, dishwashing liquid, and water. Pour the solution into a spray bottle. Spray areas where pests congregate.

Lemon Verbena Solution

   2 tablespoons lemon verbena
   1 cup alcohol
   2 tablespoons lemon-scented dishwashing
   liquid

Add lemon verbena to the alcohol. Let
steep for 2 weeks and strain. Add the
lemon-scented dishwashing liquid. Pour
this into a spray bottle and mist areas
where you see pests. This also works on
roaches.

To Get Rid of Ants

Cayenne Pepper: Sprinkle cayenne pepper
around areas where ants are usually seen.
Cinnamon: Sprinkle powdered cinnamon
where you usually find ants.
Spearmint: Place sprigs of spearmint in
areas where you find ants.

PLANT & GARDEN SPRAYS

Natural Fertilizers

Plant Fertilizer Manure

  cow and chicken manure
  water

To a 5-gallon (20-liter) bucket, add 1 gallon (4 liters) of fresh cow manure and chicken manure. Let the mix soak for 30 days in a warm spot; a greenhouse is ideal. Pour off the liquid into a large tub and add enough water to make a weak solution that's light brown. Use this to water plants up to three times a year.

  This is good for fertilizing houseplants and outside plants. It is especially good to use when you plant vegetables. This is also helpful for plants right before they bloom.

Coffee-Grounds Fertilizer

2 cups coffee grounds
½ cup bonemeal
½ cup wood ash

Put the coffee grounds, bonemeal, and wood ash in a plastic bucket and mix well. Sprinkle around shrubs and perennials.

Lawn Fertilizer

1 cup Epsom salts
1 cup ammonia
water

Mix the Epsom salts and ammonia in a glass jar. Seal. When ready to use, mix 2 tablespoons of this concentrate in a 2-gallon (7.6-liter) watering can. Sprinkle over the lawn. Mixed with water, this formula covers 200 sq. feet (18 sq. meters).

In the past, rather than piling up compost heaps, farmers utilized their barn cleanings on fields as a way of feeding their crops. Native Americans buried a fish each time they planted a corn seed to "feed" the corn. Today, most city-dwellers, suburbanites, and, indeed, most farmers do not have animals to supply manure for gardens. So, we bypass that process and place our kitchen scraps directly into the compost heap.

The traditional farmhouse kitchen scraps went to the chickens and hogs. Hogs especially love spoiled milk and other scraps that most other animals will not eat. Chickens eat almost anything, too. Twice a year, chicken and hog pens were cleaned out and manure was used to enrich garden soil.

Today, we add kitchen scraps to the soil and allow them to decompose. Then we add the compost to our gardens.

Weeds

Easy Weed Killer
boiling water
salt

To kill weeds in cracks of sidewalks or driveways, simply bring water to boil and pour it hot onto weeds. Or add salt to boiling water and use that. But keep the boiling water and salt away from plants you want to keep.

Natural Insecticides

Marigold & Garlic Spray
  marigold leaves and flowers
  3 to 4 mashed garlic cloves
  boiling water
  ¼ cup dishwashing liquid

Fill a Mason jar with marigold flowers and leaves and the mashed garlic cloves. Pour boiling water over the marigolds and garlic. Let cool and strain. Add the dishwashing liquid. Pour this into a spray bottle and soak down plants. This formula helps get rid of aphids, beetles, and squash bugs.

De-Bugging Spray

2 cups warm water
1 tablespoon dishwashing liquid

Mix the water and dishwashing liquid well and spray it on plants. For yards, attach a sprayer to which 1 cup of dishwashing liquid has been added. Spray grass, bushes, and plants regularly to get rid of pesky problems.

Garden Insecticide

1 tablespoon dishwashing liquid
1 cup vegetable oil

Mix the dishwashing liquid with vegetable oil. To use, add 2 teaspoons of this mixture to 1 cup of water. Spray on plants including under the leaves. Store this concentrate so that you can use it when needed. It helps protect growing vegetables.

Interplanting to Control Insects

Try planting these herbs and flowers around plants you want to protect.

Mint & Rosemary: To control aphids, plant mint or rosemary around fruit trees.

Catnip: Catnip repels the cabbage moth.

Marigolds: The Mexican bean beetle, tomato hornworm, and whiteflies all hate marigolds.

Garlic: Japanese beetles dislike garlic.

Wormwood: Slugs avoid wormwood.

Crickets & Grasshoppers Remedy

2 cups molasses
2 cups warm water

Mix 2 cups molasses with 2 cups warm water in a Mason jar. Set these in the garden as traps to get rid of crickets and grasshoppers.

Insecticide Juice

tomato leaves and stems
boiling water

Fill a Mason jar with tomato leaves and stems and pour boiling water over them and let cool. Strain. Pour the solution into a spray bottle. Spritz houseplants or outdoor plants. This natural insecticide will kill green flies, plant lice, and other pests.

Tomato Hornworm Remedy

powdered hot peppers

These green worms with white stripes feed on leaves of tomato plants and sometimes the fruit, as well as on eggplant, potatoes, and peppers. Get rid of them by drying some hot peppers.

Wear protective glasses and cover mouth and nose. Put peppers into a blender or food processor and grind them to powder. Wear gloves and sprinkle this powder onto the plants.

Apple Maggot Trap

   molasses
   water
   yeast

Apple maggots are small white worms that look like maggots; they cause rotten apples, plums, cherries. To get rid of them, use clean pint (500-ml) Mason jars half full with a mixture of molasses and water. Add a little yeast. Wrap string or wire around each jar and hang the jars in fruit-tree limbs. You'll trap small apple maggots before they get a chance to lay eggs.

Buttermilk Spray for Spider Mites

flour
buttermilk

Spider mites cause leaves on roses, ivy, and many vegetables to turn brown. They appear as tiny red dots on the leaves.

Mix flour and buttermilk to make a thickened liquid. Spray this liquid on the infested plants.

Marigold Spray for Spider Mites

4 tablespoons marigold flowers and leaves
2 cups boiling water

Make a spray with marigold tea. Use 4 tablespoons marigold flowers and leaves to 2 cups boiling water. Steep for 10 minutes. Cool; use as a spray on plants.

Snails & Slugs

Snails and slugs feed on many plants and can become a nuisance. They have soft bodies and congregate where it is dark and damp.

Salt: To rid yourself of these pests, sprinkle them with salt.

Beer: Set out a foil pie pan filled with beer.

Tobacco Tea: Spray surrounding areas with a tea made from tobacco leaves.

Cabbage Worm Remedy #1

1 cup salt
1 gallon (3.8 liters) warm water

Mix well and pour the salty water onto cabbages. Do this twice, 1 week apart, and the worms will be destroyed. You can also use this to prevent cabbage worms from destroying your cabbage.

Cabbage Worm Remedy #2

   2 tablespoons mild dishwashing liquid
   2 cups kerosene
   1½ gallons (6 liters) water

Bring soap and water to boiling, and then remove from heat and stir in the kerosene. Keep in a spray bottle to spray plants down as needed.

Cucumber & Melon-Vine Bugs

Cayenne Pepper: Dust plants with cayenne pepper in the morning before the dew has dried. Repeat once a week.

Ashes & Kerosene: To kill the striped bugs that destroy these plants, try mixing ashes with kerosene. Bury a handful of this mixture near the hill closest to the plant. This reportedly drives away bugs.

LAUNDRY

Spot & Stain Removers

Stain-Lifter for Pretreating Laundry
leftover soat bits
boiling water

You'll need a squeeze bottle like one you'd
use for dispensing honey. Gather leftover
bits of soap too small to use in the bath.
Place them in the squeeze bottle. When
the bottle is half full of soap, add boiling
water. The soap will melt into a jelly.
Shake well to mix. Use this soap to pre-
treat stains on clothing before laundering
them.

Spot & Stain Troubleshooting

White vinegar removes most stains and helps dissolve grease. You can use these spot removers on clothing, tablecloths, curtains, and other household cloth fabrics.

Coffee & Wine Stains: Blot with club soda or make a paste of water and salt and blot.

Fruit & Wine Stains: Use 1 teaspoon ammonia to ½ cup rubbing alcohol. Blot gently.

Ink Stains: Wet the stain with water. Make a paste of lemon juice and cream of tartar. Apply, let sit for 60 minutes, and wash as usual. Or dissolve the ink with glycerin and rinse.

Grease Spots: Rub a raw potato over the stain.

Delicate Fabrics: Add 1 tablespoon glycerin to ½ cup water. Mix well and use a cloth to blot the stain gently.

Old Lace & Tablecloths

Alcohol & Water Wash

water
alcohol

To bring new life to old lace and to table-cloths, in a dishpan or pail mix equal amounts of water and alcohol. Squeeze the cloth in the mixture, wring it out gently, and lay it flat to dry.

Lace Wash

1 rounded teaspoon borax
1 rounded teaspoon sugar
2 cups warm water

To launder lace, add the borax and sugar to the water. Mix. Gently squeeze the cloth in the borax-sugar water to clean it. Rinse and lay it out flat to dry.

Starch

Homemade Spray Starch

  1 cup cold water
  1 tablespoon cornstarch

Mix the water and cornstarch. Pour it into a spray bottle and keep the starch handy for ironing. Shake before using.

SOAPS

Soapmaking

Soapmaking is a traditional but necessary art that's fun to try today. You can make many different kinds of soap to suit your imagination—hard soaps, soft soaps, soaps made with different fats, soaps with varied scents and hues. Basically, all soap is made the same way by combining fat, water, and lye. The differences come from your choices of ingredients and their amounts.

If you make a large enough batch, you'll only have to make soap once a year. Then whenever you need soap, you can just raid your closet instead of going to the store to pay those high prices. Fall was a traditional soapmaking time, since butchering was done at that time and there was plenty of animal fat on hand.

Leftover soap will last years and years; in fact, the older the soap the better it lathers. You can use homemade soap to create your own dishwashing liquid and laundry soap. Look for recipes in this chapter.

You can find lard or tallow at the butcher's shop or in the meat department at some grocery stores. You can also buy lye in grocery stores.

Wood-Ash Lye

Lye wasn't always easily purchased from the local grocery in those convenient crystals. Before that consumer luxury, people in the 19th century made their own lye by leaching it from wood ashes. This wood-ash lye, known as potash, is much less caustic than the commercial kind we commonly use today. Made up mainly of potassium carbonate, potash is easy to formulate yourself, if you want to experiment. Wood-ash lye, like today's commercial lye, was used for making soap. Mixed with fat and water, it makes an everyday soap.

Making Wood-Ash Lye

You'll need a wooden bucket with a 1-inch (2.5-cm) hole in the side 1 inch (2.5 cm) up from the bottom, a medium-size crock (the kind they used to make pickles in), some hardwood ash (oak is best), and straw.

Line the bottom of the bucket with 1 to 2 inches (2.5 to 5 cm) of straw; then pack the ash tightly to fill the bucket, making a good-size depression in the middle. This depression will hold the boiling water that you'll pour on top of the ash. The crock should be positioned under the hole in the bucket to catch the liquid that will seep through. This liquid will be your lye.

Go slowly in this process. Pour more boiling water over the ash as the liquid disappears. Keep the process going; it may take several days to get the desired amount of lye. At the end of this process, you'll have homemade lye just like that which people made in earlier centuries.

Lye & Soapmaking Cautions

Be very careful and make sure that pets and children are out of the way. Also wear gloves and safety glasses. You'll want to use a utility-room sink, not your kitchen or bathroom sink. Lye is very caustic. Don't inhale fumes when mixing lye and never mix lye with hot water, since this will cause it to boil over. Pour the lye into the water rather than the other way around.

Soapmaking 1-2-3

1. In 1-gallon (4-liter) widemouthed glass jug or heatproof jar 2 quarts (2 liters) or larger, measure cold water that's 70 to 75° F (21.1 to 23.9° C). It must be this temperature. Place this in your sink.

Stir continuously with a wooden spoon and slowly add the lye. The water will heat up to over 200° F (93.3° C). Keep stirring to dissolve the lye completely. Use a glass, dairy, or soapmaking thermometer to check when the water-lye solution cools to the correct temperature in your recipe. At the same time, melt the fat on the stove in a 10- to 12-quart (10- to 12-liter) old enamel pot; use another thermometer to bring it to the correct temperature for your recipe.

2. When both the water-lye mixture and the fat are at the correct temperatures, in the sink slowly add the water-lye mixture to the fat, stirring constantly. The temperature of both the water-lye and the fat must be within 5° F (3° C) of each other. Stir constantly for 15 minutes. The liquid will be thin, but as you keep stirring, it will slowly thicken. You'll know your soap is done when it will "trace" or leave a mark when you lift your spoon. If it hasn't thickened after 15 minutes, wait another 15 minutes, and stir and test it again. Do this again until the mixture finally thickens.

When it "traces," stir in 1 to 2 tablespoons of a desired essential oil and, if you have hard water, add 2 cups of borax.

3. Pour the soap into prepared molds. Use commercial molds, wooden trays, shoe boxes, or cardboard boxes with the sides cut down. Line the molds with heavy-duty wax paper 1 inch (2.5 cm) from the top of the trays on all sides. Use tape to secure the

paper so that it doesn't move or wrinkle. Cover the soap-filled molds with a piece of wood, then with a blanket.

4. After 24 to 48 hours, don gloves to unmold the soap. Cut it into bars with a knife or use a wire to cut it just as you would cheese. Lay the soaps on brown-paper grocery sacks placed on top of plastic trash bags to air out and dry for at least 3 to 4 weeks. Or lay them out on wooden racks and shelves. After this period, store the soaps in plastic bags with "zippers" or plastic containers, or wrap them for gift-giving.

You may have a batch that doesn't turn out; the lye-water and fats may separate. When this happens, reheat the mixture to 140° F (60° C), stirring constantly. When that temperature is reached, remove from heat and stir until the mixture "traces." You can then pour it into molds again.

Classic Soaps

Basic Soap

   1 can (12 ounces or 336 g) commercial lye
   2½ cups water
   6 pounds fat or 13½ cups half beef tallow,
    half lard

Bring the lye-water to 93° F (33.8° C) and the fat to 125° F (51.7° C) before mixing them together. If you wish, you can use 6¾ cups beef tallow and 6¾ cups lard, to total 13½ cups, in place of the 6 pounds of fat. Proceed with the Soapmaking 1–2–3 directions on pp. 427–429. Heed the basic soapmaking cautions on p. 426.

This recipe makes 36 bars or about 9 pounds (4 kg).

Soap from Scratch

6 pounds wood ash
4 pounds lard
¼ pound pine resin

Mix the wood ash, lard, and pine resin.
Let sit for 5 days. Put the mixture in a 10-
gallon (38-liter) barrel and fill the barrel
with warm water. Stir the mixture with a
big stick morning and night for 10 days.
Pour the soap into prepared molds.

This pine soap recipe does not produce a
high-quality soap, but it satisfies those of
us who are curious about how American
pioneers made their soap.

Castile Soap

1 can (12 ounces or 336 g) lye
4 cups water
38 ounces (1.1 kg) good tallow
3 cups olive oil
3 cups coconut oil

Mix the lye and water. In a separate pan, mix the tallow, olive oil, and coconut oil. Bring both the lye-water mixture and the fats mixture separately to 90° F (32.2° C) before combining them. Then follow the Soapmaking 1–2–3 directions on pp. 427–429.

This recipe makes a hard, white soap.

Medicated Soap

  1 pound (0.45 kg) castile soap
  1 ounce (28 g) powdered sulfur

Grate the castile soap and melt it on top of a double boiler. Stir in the powdered sulfur. Pour this into prepared molds. Cut into bars and dry. Use this soap for sensitive skin, skin disease, or irritation.

Fancy Soaps

Soap Scent

  1 tablespoon lavender essential oil
  2 teaspoons dried rosemary
  1 teaspoon powdered cinnamon

Here's a scent combo. Mix lavender essential oil with dried rosemary and powdered cinnamon. Just add it to the almost finished basic soap recipe.

Nourishing Dry-Skin Soap

2 cups cold water
½ cup lye (commercial)
½ cup coconut oil
2½ cups vegetable shortening
½ cup sweet almond oil
½ cup castor oil
¼ cup powdered herbs (optional)
1 tablespoon essential oil(s) (optional)

Let the lye-water mixture come to 90 to 100° F (32 to 38° C). If necessary, put the jar in a pan of cold water. Melt the vegetable shortening and combine it with the coconut oil, sweet almond oil, and castor oil. Let the oil mixture cool to between 90 to 100° F (32 to 38° C). Combine the lye-water with the oils and stir until thickened. Add the powdered herbs and essential oils. Continue stirring until the mixture "traces." Pour it into prepared molds.

Glycerin Soap

1 can lye (12 to 13 ounces or 336 to 365 g)
2½ cups cold water
10 cups vegetable shortening
2 cups olive oil
1½ cups coconut oil
¾ cup glycerin
1 to 2 tablespoons essential oil(s)

Bring the lye-water mixture to 90 to 95° F
(32 to 35° C). If necessary, put the pan in
cold water to help bring down the temperature. Heat and melt the shortening, olive
oil, and coconut oil to 100 to 110° F (37 to
43° F). Pour the lye-water into the fats,
stirring constantly. Now add the glycerin.
When the mixture thickens, add the essential oils you've chosen. When the mixture
"traces," pour it into molds.

Creamy Oatmeal & Rose Soap

1 cup oatmeal
½ cup rose petals
1 cup goat's milk or half and half
1 can (12 to 13 ounces or 336 to 364 g) lye
3½ cups water
13 cups tallow or lard
1 tablespoon rosewood or rose-geranium
  essential oil

Blend the oatmeal, rose petals, and goat's milk in a blender. The mixture should be powdered.

Bring a mixture of lye and water to 96 to 98° F (35 to 37° C) and the tallow or lard (fat) to 98 to 100° F (37 to 38° C). Then combine the lye-water with the fat. When it just begins to thicken, add the goat's milk mixture and keep stirring until it "traces."

At this time, add rosewood essential oil or rose-geranium essential oil. If you feel really extravagant, add expensive rose essential oil. When ready, pour the soap into a mold 19×12½ inches (47.5×31.25 cm or rough equivalent). Cut into bars after 24 hours.

Tropical Dream Soap

1 tablespoon lemon-verbena leaves
⅓ cup boiling water
1⅓ cups grated Ivory soap
4 drops grapefruit essential oil
2 drops lemon essential oil
2 drops basil essential oil
1 drop lime essential oil
petroleum jelly

For your mold, wash an empty cardboard half-gallon (2-liter) milk carton. Cut it down to about 4 inches (10 cm) high and grease the inside with petroleum jelly.

Make strong lemon-verbena tea, using 1 tablespoon lemon-verbena leaves in ⅓ cup boiling water. Steep for 10 minutes. Strain. Put the brewed lemon-verbena tea on the stove and bring it to a boil; then reduce the heat to simmer.

Stir the grated soap into the strong lemon-verbena tea. Continue stirring until the soap melts and the mixture is well blended. Remove from heat and add the grapefruit, lemon, basil, and lime essential oils. Mix well again and pour into the mold.

Dry until firm. Age at least 1 week after removing from the mold. This recipe makes two bars.

You can use two molds from the milk carton or simply use one and cut the finished soap in half.

✿

Mint Soap Balls

   2 bags peppermint tea
   ⅓ cup boiling water
   3¼ cups grated castile soap (about 2 bars)
   3 drops peppermint essential oil

Make a strong peppermint tea, using 2 bags tea to ⅓ cup boiling water. While the peppermint tea is hot, pour it over the grated castile soap and knead. Add the peppermint essential oil and mix well. Form into balls. Let the soap balls air dry on waxed paper about 1 week.

To smooth the balls, place them under running water and rub. Let dry and store.

Chamomile Spice Soap

  4 tablespoons fresh or 2 tablespoons dried
    chamomile
  4 tablespoons warmed glycerin
  1½ cups finely grated unscented soap
  2 tablespoons honey
  4 drops chamomile essential oil
  10 drops clary-sage essential oil
  10 drops nutmeg essential oil

Add fresh or dried chamomile to the warmed glycerin. Remove from heat and cover. Let this sit overnight. Strain.

Melt the soap on top of a double boiler. Remove from heat and add the herbed glycerin. Stir in the honey and the chamomile, clary-sage, and nutmeg essential oils. Mix well. Pour into greased molds.

This recipe makes two bars.

Homemade Soap Solutions

Hand Dishwashing & Laundry Detergent

Before switching from commercial soaps, just this once, run the clothes through the wash with 1 cup baking soda and no soap to clean the fabric of residues and to prevent yellowing. After that, just add a ½ cup baking soda or borax to each wash when you add your homemade cleanser.

If you use grated soap flakes alone, it can be difficult to get the soap to dissolve completely. After doing laundry, you'll have errant soap pieces all over your clean clothes.

❧

Here are two easy recipes for hand dishwashing and for laundry detergent.

Jellied Soap

½ pound (224 g) homemade grated soap
2 quarts (1.8 liters) water
½ teaspoon sassafras or another essential oil

Grate the homemade soap. Bring 2 quarts (2 liters) of water to boil and add the soap shavings. Boil for about 10 minutes and cool.

Old recipes call for scenting the soap with oil of sassafras, but you can scent it with any essential oil you wish. Keep the jellied soap in a closed container. This makes a jellied soap you can use for both clothes washing or dishwashing.

Easy Soapy-Water Wash

3 or more soap bars
boiling water

Place a few bars of soap into a wide-mouthed ½-gallon (2-liter) jar, the kind used for canning or any heatproof jar. Pour boiling water into this and let it cool. Shake it a few times.

When you get ready to wash dishes or clothes, run the hot water. Then add some of this soapy liquid. You'll have to experiment to get the right amount of soap for what you want to accomplish.

Replace the liquid you use from the jar with more boiling water until the soap bars disappear. Then you can simply add more soap bars and begin the process again.

CANDLES & POTPOURRI

Beeswax Candles

Beeswax candles smell heavenly. They don't smoke like other waxes. When making candles, remember that a wick too narrow for your candle will cause the wax to drown the flame, and a wick too thick will smoke.

Candle Molds

Meantime, prepare your molds. Small waxed-paper cups work for votives. Cut-down milk cartons make good candle chunks. Jelly jars also work, as do commercial candle molds. Spray the molds with a cooking spray so that they come out easily.

Wicks

Make wicks by cutting the cotton wicking 3 to 4 inches (7.5 to 10 cm) longer than your mold and dipping it into the wax. Lay the wick out to cool on waxed paper. Attach tiny fishing sinkers to the bottoms or tie the string to something weighted, like metal buttons or flat washers.

❦

Preparing the Beeswax

If your beeswax is fresh from the hive and not yet cleaned, here's how to clean it. On low heat, melt the wax and add a little—not much—apple-cider vinegar and water to it. Keep the temperature at 135 to 140° F (57 to 60° C) for at least 12 hours. Maintain the temperature for 2 days, if you can.

After the 2 days, the heated wax should float to the top. The honey should make up the next layer, with dirt at the bottom. Merely skim off the beeswax and place it in another old pan.

445

Beeswax Candlemaking

Heat up the prepared beeswax to 200° F (94° C). Pour the wax into prepared molds and set your wicks in the middle, tying the tops of the wick(s) to a pencil or Popsicle stick placed over the top of the mold. This holds the wick in place in the middle of the candle. Let the candle set to harden and cool. Then trim the wicks.

Dipped Beeswax Candles

Melt your wax in a deep container and have a larger container full of ice water. Heat the wax to 200° F (94° C). Hold a length of cotton wicking in the middle. You should have about 6 to 8 inches (15 to 20 cm) of wick hanging on each end. Or decide how long you want these taper candles.

Wear long gloves so that you don't burn your fingers or arms with splashed hot wax. Now put the wick on a wooden spoon so that the wick hangs down each side. Dip the wick ends into the wax. Then dunk it into the ice water. Now dip it into the hot wax again, then into the ice water. Each time you repeat these steps, your candle will get fatter. When it is as fat as you want, hang the candles to dry and harden. Trim the wicks before you burn them.

Rolled Wax Candles

Beeswax sheets make easy rolled beeswax candles. Purchase beeswax sheets from craft shops or beekeeping suppliers. You can buy the sheets in multicolors, too. Since they are about 16 inches (40 cm) long, cut your wicking accordingly.

Place the wax sheets in a warm place—80 to 85° F (26 to 30° C)—so that they will be pliable. Cut the sheet on an angle so that the top edge slants down a little for three or four rolls. Place your wick on the high edge and begin rolling tightly. Use your warm fingers to press the edge to seal the last roll, and it's finished.

Paraffin, Tallow & Other Candles

Paraffin Candles

  paraffin
  beeswax
  candle dyes or crayons
  stearic acid
  essential oils (optional)

Paraffin candles are less expensive to make than beeswax candles. You can add essential oils for scent after removing the paraffin from the heat. Beeswax candles can be scented, too, but you may not want to scent them since they have a sweet, natural scent all their own.

To make the candles last longer, you may want to mix half paraffin and half beeswax. That will make a superior candle. Or if you're making tapers, make your last three or four dips beeswax so that the outer layer is beeswax and the inner layer is paraffin. Candles kept in the refrigerator reportedly burn longer.

When melting the wax, you may want to use a coffee can with a lip bent into the top rim for a pouring spout. Use oven mitts to handle it. Place the coffee can in a pot with 6 to 8 inches (15 to 20 cm) of water that you bring to simmer. Melt the wax slowly on low heat.

For every 2 pounds (56 g) of wax (paraffin and beeswax), add ⅓ cup of stearic acid after it is melted. Also add any coloring agents—candle dyes or crayons—then.

You can buy candle dyes from candle supply companies or shops that sell beekeeping equipment. If you don't want to use candle dyes, add one or two crayons. You can get a wide variety of colors from crayons, and they don't cost much.

Tallow Candles

2 pounds (0.9 kg) deer, goat, or beef tallow
beeswax (optional)
⅓ cup alum or stearic acid
string

You'll need some tallow (fat). Beef tallow is okay, but deer or goat tallow makes a better candle. Melt and strain the tallow twice through cheesecloth. You might even want to just skim the fat off the top for the best-quality, clearest fat. Add some beeswax, if you have it. You'll also want to add alum or stearic acid since that helps harden the candle. About 2 pounds (0.9 kg) of fat makes about 12 candles.

❦

Emergency Candle
  mullein leaf
  bacon grease
  jar lid
  sand

If you are out camping or just need an emergency light, here's a recipe for you. Dip a mullein leaf into bacon grease and roll it into a tight stick. Let the grease cool until the leaf is stiff. Then put this mullein stick in an empty jar lid that's turned up.

Heap sand around the bottom to make it stand upright. Light the mullein leaf and you'll have a rustic candle.

Mullein used to be called hag's taper. Ancient Romans dipped mullein flower stalks into tallow to make torches.

Decorated & Holiday Candles

Decorated Candle

  large round candle
  hair spray
  white glue
  potpourri
  cinnamon
  ground cloves
  wax

Use a large round candle. Spray the sides with hair spray and let them dry. Next apply glue all around the sides but not on the candle's top or bottom. Have a bowl filled with the potpourri of your choice. Cinnamon and ground cloves in the mix work especially well, as do other potpourri ingredients. Let the glue dry overnight.

The next day, set a coffee can in boiling water. Inside the can, melt some wax at 185 to 200° F (85 to 94° C). Have a cold-water dipping pan handy.

Put a few drops of essential oil all around and on the potpourri that's glued to the candle. Tie a string to the wick of the candle and dip the candle all the way into the wax so that the potpourri will be covered. Dip in the water and drain. Repeat the procedure.

You'll be able to see the potpourri through the wax. As the candle burns, it will release a delicious aroma. Use this decorated candle to dress up a table or give it as a gift. It emits a pleasing, spicy scent.

❧

Metal Candleholder

tin or metal can

With tin snips, cut away the side of a tin or metal can, leaving one side on and a 1-inch (2.5-cm) rim up from the bottom. You can cut the can in decorative shapes, if you wish. Next, punch a hole in the top of the remaining can wall and you'll be able to hang your candleholder.

Place a candle in the bottom of the can, and the tin side behind it will reflect the light out wonderfully. Hang the metal candleholder on a wall from a hook.

Party Candle Luminaries

glass jars
wire
sand

Use glass jars the size to fit your candle.
Jelly jars work well for votives, and pint
(480- to 500-ml) or Mason jars work for
larger candles. Twist wire around the rim
of the jar to make a handle like a bucket.
Add 1 to 2 inches (2.5 to 5 cm) of sand in
the bottom of the jar and set the candle
down into it. Now light and hang the jars
in the yard for parties and nighttime bar-
becues. The jars keep the candles from
blowing out or being knocked over.

Bug-Proofing: Put a few drops of citronella essential oil on the melted wax near
the wick. Stay away from the flame; the
essential oil is volatile.

Holiday Candle-Bag Luminaries

small paper bags or plastic milk jugs
candles
sand

These candleholders decorate your entryway for holiday parties and special occasions in a festive way. Neatly roll down the tops of brown or white paper lunch sacks several times. If you wish, cut out holiday designs on each bag, like a jack-'o-lantern face or snowflake. After you have cut out the design, you'll want to tape a piece of thin paper over the cutouts to prevent the wind from blowing out the candle.

Place 3 to 6 inches (8 to 16 cm) of sand in the bottom of each bag, and nestle a candle down in the middle. The bag height must be at least 3 or 4 inches (7.5 or 10 cm) higher than that of the candle.

Now line the walkway up to you door and at dusk, light your candles.

If you collect plastic milk jugs, you can use them instead of the paper bags. Rinse the jugs well and cut off their tops. Make the milk-jug luminaries all the same height, well above that of the candle. Add sand to the bottom and put the candle down in the center, supported by the sand.

These can brighten a path for Halloween trick-or-treaters to your door. They also work well around Christmas and can sit along a driveway in snow. Some neighborhoods use them Christmas Eve for a kind of light-up night.

Since these bags contain burning candles, use them with care.

Dry Potpourri

People once covered floors with dried, scented herbs to mask unpleasant odors in the home. The practice of herb strewing began long before cleanliness was considered next to godliness. Later, herbal scents were used medicinally to "drive out" evil spirits, that is, germs.

Potpourris freshen rooms naturally, just as strewn herbs do. Potpourris are a more sophisticated and less messy expression of herb strewing. Rose petals are the most popular ingredient in traditional potpourris and may indeed have been the first potpourri ingredient ever used.

Dry the herbs and flowers for these recipes on screens or newspapers in a warm, darkened room out of direct sunlight until completely dry. For finished potpourri, use translucent or transparent containers with lids you can remove as you wish.

Old-Fashioned Potpourri Mix

2 cups dried rose petals
1 cup dried lavender buds
1 cup dried rose-geranium leaves
½ cup dried rosemary
1 tablespoon crushed cinnamon
1 tablespoon whole cloves
1 tablespoon nutmeg
3 tablespoons powdered orrisroot
2 tablespoons gum benzoin
8 drops rose or rosewood essential oil
5 drops lavender essential oil

Mix the rose petals, lavender buds, rose-geranium leaves, rosemary, crushed cinnamon, whole cloves, and nutmeg. For a fixative, add the powdered orrisroot and gum benzoin. Add the rose or rosewood essential oil and the lavender essential oil. Enclose all these ingredients in a tightly closed jar or box. Open for a half hour to scent the room.

Fresh & Fruity Potpourri

plum or peach stones
4 cups dried rose petals
1 cup dried chamomile
1 cup dried sweet woodruff
½ cup lemon verbena
3 tablespoons dried, curled lemon peel
2 tablespoons coarse salt
1 tablespoon powdered benzoin gum
2 tablespoons nutmeg
8 drops lemon essential oil
10 drops chamomile essential oil

In preparation a few days before you make the potpourri, clean and dry plum, peach, or other fruit stones for decoration in the mix. Shave lemon peel into curls and dry. Mix the rose petals, chamomile, sweet woodruff, lemon verbena, lemon peel, coarse salt, benzoin gum, nutmeg, lemon essential oil, and chamomile essential oil. Add the fruit stones.

Allow the mixture to set in a closed container for several weeks to let the fragrance blend. Put the potpourri in decorative jars, ready to use.

The coarse salt acts as a preservative and the benzoin gum acts as a fixative.

Fresh-as-Outdoors Potpourri

   1 cup granulated sugar
   3 tablespoons real maple syrup
   2 cups green, fresh pine needles
   1 cup cedar chips
   1 cup small pinecones
   1 cup dried sweet woodruff
   10 drops rosewood essential oil
   8 drops sandalwood essential oil

Mix the sugar and maple syrup well. Let it sit out until the sugary texture is dry. Add a little more white sugar if the mixture seems too wet. The sugar acts as a preservative. To this sugar add the pine needles, cedar chips, pinecones, sweet woodruff, rosewood essential oil, and sandalwood essential oil. Blend well.

Put the potpourri in a closed container for 3 weeks. Then you can transfer it to one or more decorative containers or open dishes. Set them out to scent a room.

Christmas Potpourri

1 cup wood shavings
2 cups dried rosemary
2 cups green pine needles
½ cup dried, curled orange peel
½ cup small pinecones
1 tablespoon powdered cinnamon
1 tablespoon whole nutmeg
1 tablespoon whole cloves
10 drops frankincense essential oil

8 drops sandalwood essential oil
6 drops pine essential oil
6 drops orange essential oil
2 or more cinnamon sticks (optional)
pine sprig (optional)
ribbon (optional)

Prepare curls of orange peel and dry them for a few days. Mix the wood shavings, rosemary, pine needles, dried orange peel, pinecones, cinnamon, nutmeg, and cloves. Add the frankincense, sandalwood, pine, and orange essential oils. Blend well using a wooden spoon. Put the spice mixture in a closed container and let sit for 4 weeks.

Add broken cinnamon sticks to the potpourri mixture, if you wish. Or, for decoration, tie two cinnamon sticks together with ribbon and a pine sprig. Put the decoration on top of the potpourri or tie it around the neck of an attractive jar.

Old-Fashioned Rose Potpourri

4 cups rose petals
1 tablespoon orrisroot
2 tablespoons sliced ginger root
1 teaspoon aniseed

Pick the roses when almost fully open or three-fourths the way to full bloom. Dry them completely on a screen or newspaper. To the rose petals, add the orrisroot, ginger root, and aniseed. Mix well and put the potpourri mixture in a dish with a lid or any type of pretty container. Let the mixture age for 4 weeks.

Moist Potpourri

This method produces the strongest aroma, although the look and color won't be as pretty as that of dried potpourris. For this reason, you may wish to place these potpourris in opaque containers.

Moist Rose Jar

rose petals
coarse noniodized salt
6 to 8 drops rose essential oil (optional)

Gather rose petals. Dry the petals about 2 to 3 days until leathery. Into a nice wide-mouthed jar with a lid, put ½ inch (1.25 cm) of rose petals; then sprinkle ¼ inch (0.6 cm) of coarse salt over them. Repeat this layering until the jar is three-fourths full. Press the flowers down with a mallet and weight it with a saucer and rock. Stir each day for 10 days. Break the chunks up and stir in 6 to 8 drops of rose essential oil to make the scent stronger.

Store the rose potpourri in decorative containers with lids. Open the rose jar for a half hour to scent a room. This traditional moist potpourri will keep for years.

Moist Lavender Jar

  4 cups dried lavender buds
  coarse noniodized salt
  2 teaspoons fruit brandy or vanilla or
   lavender essential oil

Layer ½ inch (1.25 cm) of lavender buds
and ¼ inch (0.6 cm) of salt. Pour about 2
teaspoons of fruit brandy over all. Instead
of the fruit, add vanilla or lavender essential oil, if you wish.

  Close the jar. For 10 days, stir once each
day. Put the lavender potpourri in decorative containers and close them for 3 weeks.
Then use the lavender jar(s) as you wish.

Moist Woodland Scent

1 cup fresh thyme
1 cup fresh rosemary
1 tablespoon powdered cloves
6 to 8 drops eucalyptus essential oil
coarse, noniodized salt
⅔ cup brandy

Mix the thyme, rosemary, and cloves well. Add the eucalyptus essential oil. Place ½ inch (1.25 cm) of this mixture in the bottom of a jar. Layer that with coarse salt. Keep adding the layers until the jar is three-fourths full. Pour ⅔ cup (wineglass) of brandy over it. Let it sit for 2 weeks, stirring once each day.

Put this mixture in decorative jars with lids for another 2 weeks. After the mixture steeps for this time, you can open the jar a half hour at a time to scent the room.

When your household has colds or flus, this invigorating scent is good for everyone. It disinfects the air.

Herb Disks, Balls & Pomanders

Fruit Pomanders

   orange or lemon
   whole cloves
   1 tablespoon cinnamon
   1 tablespoon nutmeg
   1 tablespoon powdered cloves
   1 tablespoon orrisroot
   3 drops orange or lemon essential oil
   ribbon

Fruit pomanders impart an especially pleasing scent during holidays. Take a fresh orange or lemon. Push whole cloves into the skin over most of the fruit. Leave a little skin clear so that you can tie a ribbon around the orange or lemon later to hang it. Roll the fruit in a spice mixture of cinnamon, nutmeg, powdered cloves, orris-root, and orange or lemon essential oil.

Wrap the spiced fruit loosely in news-paper and let it dry completely for 3 to 4 weeks.

Now tie on a pretty ribbon with a small bow. Hang this from Christmas trees, in closets, or anywhere you wish to impart a spicy scent. These fruit pomanders have the added advantage of repelling bugs.

Cinnamon-Herb Disks

1 cup cinnamon
¼ cup powdered lavender or another herb
6 to 8 drops lavender essential oil
4 to 6 tablespoons white glue
about 1 cup water
lavender buds or other herb (for decoration)

Mix the cinnamon, lavender essential oil, and the powdered lavender or herb you've chosen with 4 tablespoons white glue. Only use enough of the water to make a flexible dough you can work; add more dry mix if the dough is too wet. Cover the bowl and refrigerate for 2 to 3 hours.

Knead until smooth. Sprinkle cinnamon on your work surface and roll the dough out as you would cookie dough.

Cut into shapes with a cookie cutter. Christmas tree or heart-shaped cutters work well. Punch holes in the tops with toothpicks so that you can hang them. Bake these herb disks in a very low oven for 1½ hours to 2 hours or until dry. Cool.

Run a line of glue around the edge of the "cookie," or disk. Sprinkle on lavender buds or another dried herb so that it will stick to the glue. Let it dry completely.

Use a pretty ribbon to make a bow and hanger. Hang these cinnamon-herb disks anywhere to freshen and impart fragrance. If you hang them in windows in the winter, heat from the sun will release the cinnamon-herb fragrance into the air.

Spice Balls

½ cup raisins
¼ cup powdered nutmeg
½ cup powdered cinnamon
¼ teaspoon sandalwood essential oil
½ teaspoon frankincense essential oil
¼ teaspoon lavender essential oil
½ cup or more red wine
powdered benzoin

Mix the raisins, nutmeg, and cinnamon. Add the sandalwood, frankincense, and lavender essential oils and the red wine. Mix well and make 1-inch (2.5-cm) balls. Roll these balls in powdered benzoin. Dry for 3 weeks or until firm. As they age, the scent improves and strengthens.

Place these spice balls in drawers and closets. You could also heap a few balls in a small crystal bowl in bathroom. Another good place is in your car. Use anywhere!

Rose & Rosary

The aromatic creation of rose beads is an ancient art passed down to us through the ages. Early European Christians considered the rose a symbol of faith. The rose soon became strongly connected with early martyrs and saints and especially with the Virgin Mary. The white rose came to symbolize the Virgin's purity, while the red rose came to mean the tears she shed which turned blood-red. Even to this day, many miraculous sightings of the Virgin are connected with the rose scent.

Beads made from the petals of this sacred flower captured its scent and allowed it to be enjoyed for years. The beads strung into necklaces eventually came to be known as the rosary, which provides a way of counting prayers and acts as a reminder of the sacred quality of the scent of the rose.

Fragrant Rose Beads

1 cup fresh rose petals
30 drops white glue
8 to 10 drops rose or other essential oil
dental floss or fishing line
string or wire

Purée the rose petals or mash them into a liquid pulp. In a bowl, mix the pulp and the white glue. Add rose or another essential oil to improve the fragrance. Roll the fragrant mixture of rose petals and glue into beads. Add more white glue if necessary to make the pulp the right consistency.

Make the beads a little larger than you'd like since they shrink as they dry. With needle and fishing line or dental floss, string the beads and stretch the line to dry for 4 to 5 days. Move the beads once a day to keep them loose.

When the beads are finished, tie the string to make a scented necklace to wear. You can use string or wire for the finished necklace, if you like. Don't allow this necklace to get wet. You can also use these beads to scent linens. Traditional rosary beads were once made this way.

Substitutions: You can use another fragrant herb and essential oil—like peppermint, lavender, or lemon verbena—for the rose petals and rose essential oil.

❦

Beeswax Rose Beads

½ cup beeswax
about 1½ cup minced rose petals
10 to 15 drops rose essential oil
dental floss
wire or string

Melt the beeswax over low heat. Add 1½ cups minced rose petals or enough to form a wax paste. Add 10 to 15 drops rose essential oil. While the wax is warm, form beads and string them with dental floss. Let them harden. You can then use wire or string to string the beads.

ROOM SPRAYS

Air Fresheners & Scents

Caution: Exercise care with these room sprays. Don't let children handle them. Keep the mist off wooden furniture. Also don't let the spray get on the skin or in anyone's face. Keep them away from pets.

Heavy-Duty Room Spray
  2 cups vodka
  1 cup crushed bay leaves
  ½ cup dried sage leaves

Mix the bay leaves and sage leaves in the vodka. Let the mixture steep in a sunny window for 1 week. Strain and pour the mixture into a spray bottle. Mist the air as needed.

Lavender Car Freshener

1 tablespoon dried lavender
¼ cup boiling water
¼ cup witch hazel
½ teaspoon lemon-verbena essential oil
¼ teaspoon castor oil

Make strong lavender tea using 1 tablespoon lavender with ¼ cup boiling water. Let steep for 10 minutes. Strain. Add the witch hazel, lavender tea, lemon-verbena essential oil, and castor oil and mix well. Shake before using. Mist as needed.

Pour the mixture into small spray bottles with caps. Leave a bottle of the freshener in the car so that you can use it on occasion. It will freshen the car and rid it of smoky smells.

You can substitute concentrated lemon juice for lemon-verbena essential oil.

Cinnamon Spice Spray

　1 cup vodka
　8 whole cloves
　2 broken cinnamon sticks
　6 to 8 eucalyptus leaves

To the vodka, add the cloves, cinnamon
sticks, and eucalyptus leaves. Let the mixture steep in a sunny window for 2 weeks.
Strain. Bottle in a spray bottle.

　Use the mist to deodorize and freshen
rooms.

　Substitutions: You can substitute ¼ cup
of another herb for the eucalyptus leaves.

Mint Room Freshener

2 tablespoons peppermint
½ cup boiling water
4 tablespoons rubbing alcohol
10 drops peppermint essential oil
10 drops spearmint essential oil
1 full dropper cold-pressed, cold-processed
   castor oil

Make strong peppermint tea with 2 tablespoons peppermint and ½ cup boiling water. Steep for 10 minutes. Mix the peppermint tea, alcohol, and the peppermint and spearmint essential oils. Add the castor oil and mix well. Shake before using. Pour the mixture into a spray bottle.

When the mood strikes, mist rooms. This mist is cooling on hot summer days. Be sure to keep the spray away from wooden furniture. Don't let the spray get in anyone's face or land near pets.

Fresh Flowers Room Scent

⅔ cup vodka
¼ cup distilled water
20 drops jasmine essential oil
15 drops bergamot essential oil
6 to 8 drops rose or rose-geranium essential oil

Mix the vodka and water. Add the jasmine, bergamot, and rose or rose-geranium essential oils. Pour the mixture into a spray bottle and use it to mist rooms.

This scent is especially nice for romantic evenings.

Bathroom Fresheners

Sometimes the bathroom is the hardest room in the house to keep fresh-smelling. Here are some easy tricks. Place a few drops of the essential oils your choice on cotton balls and place them in the middle of the toilet-paper roll, inside the cardboard roll. Each time you use it, the fresh scent will be released. You'll have to refresh the roll every other day.

To scent towels, put a few drops of essential oil on a terry-cloth rag and place it in the dryer with a load of towels. The towels will come out nicely scented, and if placed in the bathroom, they will impart a pleasing scent to the air.

Long-Lasting Scent Gel

2 cups water
4 packets or 4 tablespoons unflavored gelatin
3 drops red food coloring
1 teaspoon peppermint or cinnamon essential oil

Bring 1 cup of water to boil. Pour the
water over the gelatin; stir until it is dissolved. Add 1 cup of cold water, food coloring, and the peppermint or cinnamon
essential oil. Pour this gelatin mixture into
flat tins or empty baby-food jars.

To scent a closet or room, remove the lid
of the tin or jar, and place the jar or tin in
an inconspicuous place. This scent gel
works nicely in a bathroom.

Carpet Fresheners

Tea-Tree Carpet Freshener

  4 cups baking soda
  30 drops tea-tree essential oil
  10 drops lavender essential oil

Prepare the carpet freshener by mixing the baking soda, tea-tree essential oil, and lavender essential oil. Test a small, hidden part of the carpet for color changes before using.

  Sprinkle this freshener sparingly on carpets and upholstery. Let it sit for 30 minutes and vacuum the powder up.

Potpourri Carpet Freshener

½ cup powdered potpourri
1 cup cornstarch

Powder the potpourri. Mix the potpourri and cornstarch. Sprinkle this powder over the carpet and vacuum after 30 minutes.

❧

Removing Pet Odors from Carpets

baking soda or white vinegar

Blot the fresh stain with a cloth soaked in baking soda. You can also use a cloth soaked in white vinegar.

Other Odors

Skunky Odor Remedy
  vinegar or tomato juice

For those unexpected run-ins with wildlife,
you need a remedy. For clothes, soak them
in vinegar for several hours; then wash as
usual. You may have to repeat this several
times.

  For dogs that have a stinky problem, as
well as humans, pour cans of tomato juice
over the fur or skin and hair and soak well;
then shampoo. Vinegar will also work.

Kitchen Odors

2 cups water
½ cup baking soda
30 drops tea-tree essential oil

Mix the water with the baking soda. Add the tea-tree essential oil. Use this disinfectant to sponge down countertops and refrigerators.

Natural Lemon Cleanser

lemon
water

Use a one-to-one solution of water and concentrated lemon juice. This will banish strong onion smells as well as fishy smells.

SCENT BAGS

Also called sachets or sweet bags, scent bags were very popular in the 19th and early 20th centuries for repelling damaging insects and adding scents. It was easy to tuck them into drawers, slip them into pockets or pillows, or place them in cupboards, closets, and trunks.

Scent bags are easy to make. Sew pockets from rectangles of cloth, and either tie the bundles with ribbon, making a loop to hang them, or simply sew them closed. If tied, the pouch can be refreshed. If you sew it closed, you'll have to throw the whole bundle out when the fragrance is gone.

Lavender Sachets

1 cup cornstarch
1 tablespoon coarse noniodized salt
1 tablespoon (½ ounce or 14 g) orrisroot
4 to 6 drops lavender essential oil
½ cup lavender buds

Mix the cornstarch, coarse salt, orrisroot, lavender essential oil, and lavender buds. Place the lavender mixture in little bags and decorate them with lace or with sprigs of dried lavender.

Strawberry Sweet Bags

½ cup dried strawberries
¼ cup dried rose petals
¼ cup baby powder
¼ cup dried sweet woodruff
1 tablespoon coarse noniodized salt

Chop the dried strawberries. Mix the dried strawberries, rose petals, baby powder, sweet woodruff, and coarse salt well. Put the strawberry potpourri in little lacy bags.

Rose Sachets

½ cup dried rose petals or buds
½ cup cornstarch
10 to 15 drops clove essential oil
1 tablespoon orrisroot

Mix the rose petals or buds, cornstarch, clove essential oil, and orrisroot well. Place the mixture in little bags. Decorate these sachets with a ribbon and a dried rose bud.

Remembrance of Violets

½ cup cornstarch
1 tablespoon coarse noniodized salt
1 tablespoon orrisroot
½ cup dried rose petals
20 drops jasmine essential oil
5 drops rose essential oil

Mix the cornstarch, coarse salt, orrisroot, rose petals, jasmine essential oil, and rose essential oil well. Put the mixture into little bags and tie them with violet-colored ribbons. Although there are no violets in this recipe, this combination of herbs and essential oils mimics the smell of violets. Violet essential oil is generally unavailable on the market.

Special Cautions

These herbal home remedies use largely "natural" ingredients and are, on the whole, safer to use than most commercial products.

However, exercise care when using them since all ingredients may not agree with you. Check for allergies and immediately discontinue use of a preparation if you have an allergic reaction—runny nose, hives, skin rash, redness, nausea, headache, rapid heart beat, or changes in temperament.

Do not take more than the recommended dose, and avoid overdoing it by taking multiple remedies. Do not assume that if a little is good then more is better. Some remedies may not be recommended for children, pregnant women, or the seriously ill, frail, elderly, or those on medication(s). Consult a physician for serious illnesses.

Essential oils are highly concentrated and should be used with care and diluted. Do not take them orally; use only as directed. With St.-John's-wort, avoid exposure to sun since it can be phototoxic and cause sun damage to eyes, which may eventually result in cataracts. Citrus essential oils, like lemon, orange, and mandarin, also cause sun sensitivity.

Tobacco has been linked with cancer, tumors, and cardiovascular disease. Cayenne pepper and capsicum may cause arthritislike symptoms in people who are allergic to them.

Use only cold-pressed, cold-processed castor oil; never heat or warm it. Castor oil must only be used topically, not internally, except as a purgative and then in very small amounts and only as directed. The seeds of castor beans are poisonous, although the oil reportedly is not.

Beauty and luxury supplies in this book avoid the many dyes, perfumes, stabilizers, and fillers found in many commercial cosmetics and skin treatments. Use them only as directed, topically. Check skin or nose for allergic reactions.

Discontinue use if a particular recipe doesn't agree with you.

These house and garden supplies are safer than most commercial products. It's best to wear gloves, especially if you have sensitive skin; some may irritate skin or eyes. Use sprays well away from anyone's face. Avoid breathing in fumes. Do not mix bleach and ammonia, since together they produce toxic fumes. Keep house and garden products away from children and pets. Heed all soapmaking cautions on p. 426.

Note that some herbs, essential oils, and "natural" ingredients that are safe for humans may be unsafe for pets. Cats and dogs do not respond well to tea-tree essential oil. Make sure to use only minimum dosages; a little goes a long way. Willow, yarrow, aspirin, and other herbs containing salicylates can be fatal to cats.

Use these homemade remedies only as directed. Note the shelf life for the recipe. Dispose of products that appear to have gone bad.

METRIC EQUIVALENTS

Liquid & Capacity
100 drops = ⅕ teaspoon
1 teaspoon = 5 milliliters
1 tablespoon = 3 teaspoons = 15 milliliters
2 tablespoons = 1 ounce = 30 milliliters
½ cup = 4 fluid ounces = 120 milliliters
1 cup = 8 fluid ounces = 240 milliliters
2 cups = 1 pint = 480 milliliters
2 pints = 32 fluid ounces = 1 quart = 0.9 liter
4 quarts = 1 gallon = 3.8 liters
Weight
1 ounce = 28 grams
16 ounces = 1 pound = 454 grams
2.2 pounds = 1 kilogram
Length
1 inch = 2.5 centimeters
12 inches = 30 centimeters = 1 foot
1 yard = 36 inches = 0.9 meter
39 inches = 1 meter

INDEX

496

497

510

511